Precision Healthcare: Patient Care, Decision Tools, Wearables, Legal and Ethical Issues

Edited by

Neeraj Gupta
Panipat Institute of Engineering and Technology
Samalkha, Panipat, Haryana
India

Abdelhameed Ibrahim
Faculty of Engineering, Design and Information & Communications Technology (EDICT), School of ICT
Bahrain Polytechnic, Isa Town, Bahrain

Bhavesh Vyas
NORMI Research Foundation
Gurugram, India

&

Shobhna Jeet
School of Legal Studies, K R Mangalam University
Gurugram, India

Precision Healthcare: Patient, Care, Decision Tools, Wearables Legal and Ethical Issues

Editors: Neeraj Gupta, Abdelhameed Ibrahim, Bhavesh Vyas and Shobhna Jeet

ISBN (Online): 979-8-89881-351-2

ISBN (Print): 979-8-89881-352-9

ISBN (Paperback): 979-8-89881-353-6

Published by Bentham Science Publishers Pte. Ltd. Singapore,

in collaboration with Eureka Conferences, USA.

First published in 2025.

Bentham Science Publishers Pte. Ltd.
No. 9 Raffles Place
Office No. 26-01
Singapore 048619
Singapore
Email: subscriptions@benthamscience.net

BENTHAM SCIENCE

CONTENTS

FOREWORD

As a senior pharmacologist with teaching experience of more than 38 years in the field of Healthcare, Management of Diseases, Quality of Life, Precision Medicines and Applications in clinical services, I believe that the book titled "Navigating Precision Healthcare: Patient Care, Decision Tools, Wearables, and the Legal-Ethical Landscape" will play an important role in teaching and learning of the students of health sciences, computer science with specialisation in Machine Learning and Artificial Intelligence.

The editor's acumen and knowledge in the fields of machine learning, computer science, and legal studies will provide a cutting-edge perspective in the book, offering insights from experts in medicine, technology, ethics, and law. Precision healthcare represents a paradigm shift in the way patient care is delivered, incorporating personalized treatment plans, advanced decision-making tools, especially in anti-cancer therapy.

In this book, the editors' aim is to provide healthcare professionals, researchers, policymakers, and patients with a deep understanding of the opportunities and challenges presented by precision healthcare. The enlisted chapters cover a wide range of topics, from the latest advancements in precision medicine to ethical considerations of using patient data in decision-making. The proposed book also delves into the legal implications of implementing precision healthcare practices, offering guidance on how to navigate this rapidly evolving landscape.

I hope that this book will serve as a valuable resource for anyone interested in the future of healthcare delivery. We believe that by exploring the combination of patient care, decision tools, wearables, and the legal and ethical landscape, we can collectively work towards a more personalized, efficient, and ethical healthcare system.

Arun Garg
MVN University, Palwal, Haryana, India
Indian Pharmacy Graduates' Association, India

PREFACE

Precision healthcare, or personalized healthcare, is a medical approach tailored to a person's healthcare depending upon their genetics, environment, and lifestyle factors. Based on the parameters collected through sensors such as wearables, timely intervention can be tailored to safeguard patients even if they are not under the direct supervision of a medical practitioner. Precision healthcare encompasses a broader scope, covering genomics, precision medicine, machine learning algorithms, large language models, big data analytics to support clinical decisions and documentation, various aspects of patient care, and precise decision-making based on radiology through the use of computer vision. Maintaining and respecting patient's data privacy and security is essential. The regulatory framework and law must be in tandem with ever-changing technology. Precision healthcare represents a significant shift towards individualized healthcare, aiming to improve outcomes and reduce costs in the long run. This book is an effort to bring relevant literature on healthcare in one place for use by academics, researchers, medical practitioners, and legal practitioners.

This book explores the concepts and techniques of precision healthcare, a promising and flourishing frontier in healthcare. Precision healthcare is a multidisciplinary field that draws work from machine learning, the Internet of Things, databases, statistics, information retrieval, pattern recognition, oncology, and knowledge-based systems. This book offers comprehensive information on various aspects of healthcare. The contents of this book will facilitate the reader's understanding of what is necessary in their respective fields. We aim to present an overall understanding of topics concerning precision healthcare from the students' perspectives, introduce the techniques and tools developed to facilitate healthcare operations, AI tools concerning oncology to enable researchers, complex legal frameworks and their implications, and discuss research directions. This book will encourage people from diverse backgrounds and experiences to share their thoughts, facilitating the promotion and development of this exciting and dynamic field.

The first chapter begins with outlining the foundations, challenges and AI-driven advancements shaping modern precision medicine. Chapter 2 examines how precision healthcare leverages data, AI, and collaborative innovation to deliver personalized treatments, while addressing the ethical and operational challenges that shaped its real-world adoption. Chapter 3 examines the transformative influence of the Internet of Medical Things (IoMT) on healthcare. Chapter 4 presents the IoMT-based lung disease classification to facilitate practitioners' decision-making. Chapter 5 gives insight into wearable technologies aiding the monitoring of patients' vital statistics and helping implement preventive strategies in emergencies. Chapters 6 to 8 illustrate the application of machine learning and data science in detecting and categorizing various diseases, including cardiovascular and diabetes. Chapter 9 explores the distinctive features, applications, and potential challenges associated with adopting large language models in the healthcare industry. Chapters 10 and 11 present various thoughts on ethical and legal frameworks concerning the adoption of precision healthcare technologies in the medical sector. Chapter 12 introduces the evolving field of precision healthcare and its promise for personalized, technology-driven patient care.

The editors are thankful to all the authors from various fields who have generously shared their knowledge and insights. Their contributions offer diverse perspectives, ensuring a well-rounded understanding of precision healthcare. The editors would like to express their gratitude to Prof. (Dr.) Arun Garg, Vice Chancellor, MVN University, for his valuable support. We extend our heartfelt thanks to the reviewers and our publishers for their unwavering support and dedication. This book would not have been possible without their collective efforts.

As the demand for personalized medical solutions grows, understanding the principles and applications of precision healthcare becomes increasingly essential. This book will inspire and inform, sparking new ideas and fostering advancements in precision healthcare. We invite you to explore the wealth of knowledge within these pages and join us in the journey towards a more personalized approach to medicine.

Neeraj Gupta
Panipat Institute of Engineering and Technology
Samalkha, Panipat, Haryana
India

Abdelhameed Ibrahim
Faculty of Engineering, Design and Information
& Communications Technology (EDICT), School of ICT
Bahrain Polytechnic, Isa Town, Bahrain

Bhavesh Vyas
NORMI Research Foundation
Gurugram, India

&

Shobhna Jeet
School of Legal Studies, K R Mangalam University
Gurugram, India

List of Contributors

Abdelhameed Ibrahim	Faculty of Engineering, Design and Information & Communications Technology (EDICT), School of ICT, Bahrain Polytechnic, PO Box 33349, Isa Town, Bahrain
A. Paramashivam	Rajalakshmi Engineering College, Chennai-602015, Tamil Nadu, India
Bedour Aldalbahi	School of ICT, Faculty of Engineering, Design and Information & Communications Technology (EDICT), Bahrain Polytechnic, PO Box 33349, Isa Town, Bahrain
Darshna M. Joshi	Department of Instrumentation and Control Engineering, Government Polytechnic, Ahmedabad, Gujarat, India
Garima Verma	Department of Cyber Security, School of Computer Science and Engineering, Galgotias University, Greater Noida, Uttar Pradesh, India
Harminder Kaur	Sharda University, Greater Noida, India
Komal	Department of Law, Gurugram University, Gurugram, India
Mohammed Aleemuddin Naveed	Department of Respiratory Medicine, Princess Esra Hospital, Deccan College of Medical Sciences, Kanchanbagh, Hyderabad 500058, Telangana, India
Mohammed Naseeruddin Mujahid	Department of Otolaryngology Princess Esra Hospital, Deccan College of Medical Sciences, Kanchanbagh, Hyderabad 500058, Telangana, India
Miryala Sai Srinivas	Kalinga Institute of Medical Sciences (KIMS), Bhubaneswar, India
Maryam Shaaban	Faculty of Engineering, Design and Information & Communications Technology (EDICT), School of ICT, Bahrain Polytechnic, PO Box 33349, Isa Town, Bahrain
Misha Bahmani	IILM Law School, IILM University, Gurugram, India
Nekul Chauhan	Biomedical Science, London Metropolitan University, London, India
Neeraj Gupta	Department of Information Technology, Panipat Institute of Engineering and Technology, Samalka, Haryana, India
Prashant Panwar	KR Mangalam University, India
Ravikant Dixit	CPJ College, Uttar Pradesh, India
Shiva Prakash	Department of ITCA, Madan Mohan Malaviya University of Technology, Gorakhpur, India
Shobhna Jeet	School of Legal Studies, K. R. Mangalam University, Gurugram, India
Sagee Geetha Sethu	Amity University, Dubai
S Adeeb Mujtaba Ali	Salar-E-Millat Sultan Salah Uddin Owaisi Central Research Laboratory for Cellular and Molecular Medicine, Princess Esra Hospital, Deccan College of Medical Sciences, Kanchanbagh, Hyderabad 500058, Telangana, India
Safia Begum	Salar-E-Millat Sultan Salah Uddin Owaisi Central Research Laboratory for Cellular and Molecular Medicine, Princess Esra Hospital, Deccan College of Medical Sciences, Kanchanbagh, Hyderabad 500058, Telangana, India

Sree Rama Chandra Murthy Dasika	Department of CSE, UCEOU, Hyderabad-500007, India
Urvinder Kaur	Department of Information Technology, Panipat Institute of Engineering and Technology, Samalka, Haryana, India
V. Kakulapati	Sreenidhi Institute of Science and Technology, Yamnampet, Hyderabad, Telangana-501301, India
Yaqoob Alhasan	Faculty of Engineering, Design and Information & Communications Technology (EDICT), School of ICT, Bahrain Polytechnic, PO Box 33349, Isa Town, Bahrain
Yogita Ambavta	Unity P.G. College, Lucknow, RR Mangalam University, India

CHAPTER 1

Precision Healthcare: Objectives, Challenges, and Solutions

V. Kakulapati[1,*], **Miryala Sai Srinivas**[2], **Sree Rama Chandra Murthy Dasika**[3] and **A. Paramashivam**[4]

[1] *Sreenidhi Institute of Science and Technology, Yamnampet, Hyderabad, Telangana-501301, India*

[2] *Kalinga Institute of Medical Sciences (KIMS), Bhubaneswar, India*

[3] *Department of CSE, UCEOU, Hyderabad-500007, India*

[4] *Rajalakshmi Engineering College, Chennai-602015, Tamil Nadu, India*

Abstract: Precision Medicine (PM) is an expanding discipline that necessitates the use of novel technologies to provide uniformity in data gathering from more than 1 million individuals and manage vast quantities of patient data. Nevertheless, ethical, social, and legal considerations, such as privacy, informed consent, and cost, present substantial obstacles. The idea requires significant government funding, amounting to millions of dollars, and must get approval from Congress over many years. Physicians and healthcare professionals must thoroughly comprehend molecular genetics and biochemistry to incorporate this technology into conventional healthcare procedures effectively. A precision health system necessitates a strategy that encompasses healthcare providers, payers, pharmaceutical firms, Information Technology (IT) businesses, employers, governments, and social groups in an interconnected manner. The system employs sensing technologies, computations, and communication to guarantee health data's security, privacy, and reliability. This chapter examines the goals, difficulties, implementations, and remedies of precision healthcare using Artificial Intelligence (AI) and Machine Learning (ML) methodologies.

Keywords: Technology, AI, Challenges, Drug, Governance, Healthcare, ML, NLP (Natural Language Processing), Objectives, Privacy, Precision health, Physicians, Security.

INTRODUCTION

PM is a branch of medicine that applies algorithmic analyses and quantitative, patient-specific data to administer the suitable medication to the correct patient at

* **Corresponding author V. Kakulapati:** Sreenidhi Institute of Science and Technology, Yamnampet, Hyderabad, Telangana-501301, India; E-mail: vldms@yahoo.com,

Neeraj Gupta, Abdelhameed Ibrahim, Bhavesh Vyas & Shobhna Jeet (Eds.)

the optimal moment [1, 2]. This method, endorsed by the United States, the GF (Gates Foundation), and the CZI (Chan Zuckerberg Initiative), has expanded its focus beyond genetics. It currently includes systems medicine, customized medicine, computational systems biomedicine, and P4 (Predictive, Preventative, customized, Participatory) medicine, and precision medicine. It encompasses a wide range of medical and physiological datasets.

The discipline of precision health focuses on identifying preclinical problems early, launching preventative measures, and evaluating disease risks at the individual level [3]. It encompasses individualized medical treatment that considers a person's distinct genetic, genomic, or omics makeup while incorporating lifestyle, social, economic, cultural, and environmental variables [4]. Precision health is more comprehensive than PM since it includes approaches to promote health and prevent diseases outside healthcare facilities. The goal is to align promotion, preventive, diagnosis, and treatment interventions with the genetic, biological, environmental, social, and behavioral factors influencing health while prioritizing the individual's needs [5]. Precision health fundamentally redirects attention from treatment to the promotion of health and the prevention of illness initiation.

Personalized Medicine (PM) is a data-driven method of treating health disorders by targeting individual genetic variations, replacing the expensive trial-and-error technique. Over the next two decades, PM will empower medical professionals to identify the most effective medication for a patient's therapy and reduce adverse side effects. Electronic health records will enable clinicians to access essential medical information instantly, while DNA sequencing will provide risk profiles for common ailments and individual susceptibility to certain disorders [6]. Integrating health-related data with gene mutations yields more accurate information for clinical implementation. Next Generation Sequencing (NGS) has decreased the expenses of sequencing a whole genome. At the same time, smart wearable devices will gather data to be stored in a unified database that combines genetic, metabolic, and lifestyle information. Nevertheless, PM's primary obstacle to materializing is the presence of economic, behavioral, or systemic elements.

Providing a more precise approach to the avoidance, analysis, and treatment of illness is the objective of the Precision Healthcare initiative. Conventional medical therapies have been developed to provide a “one-size-fits-all” technique. However, even though these therapies could be successful for some people, the goal of precision healthcare is to make the process of diagnosing a disease or sickness, as well as the treatment, remedies, and prevention of disease or illness, more individualized, proactive, predictive, and accuracy-oriented [7]. The fundamental objective of precision healthcare is to enhance clinical outcomes for individual patients by employing exact therapy targeting. This is accomplished by using genetic, biomarker, phenotypic, or psychological features that differentiate a specific patient from others with similar clinical presentations. Precision healthcare aims to ensure that appropriate therapies are administered to the relevant patients at the proper time (shown in Fig. **1**).

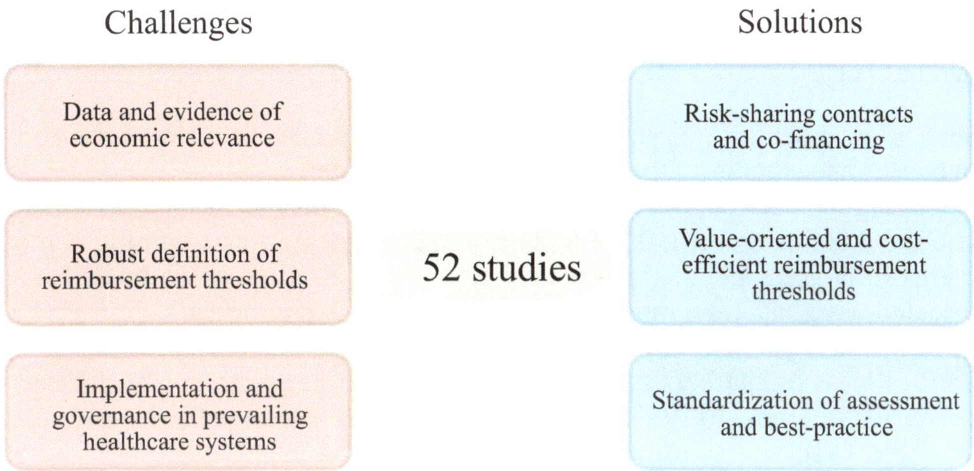

Fig. (1). Integration of personalized medicine in healthcare systems [8].

A health technology's economic case is established by contrasting its price and potential health risks with alternatives. By capitalizing on the variability among individual patients, PM has the potential to enhance cost-effectiveness. Nevertheless, the lack of clinical and economic data, as well as the reliance on assumptions, might make demonstration difficult. Prioritizing decision-makers' needs early may enhance the generation of evidence for resource allocation decisions. The economic rationale for PM may be progressively refined to minimize ambiguity [9].

The World Economic Forum's PM Programme aims to establish policy frameworks, advance societal advantages, and mitigate dangers using inventive collaborations, standards, and support models [10].

Numerous impediments hinder precision medicine, including the extensive data requirements, the necessity for secrecy and concealment, and the potential for data corruption due to noise. The data processing method currently takes 26 hours, which is too long for critical care decision-making. Assessing the accuracy of data is also tricky. Capacity development is crucial, especially in educating healthcare professionals and utilizing modern AI, machine learning, and laboratory apparatus. The focus on precision-based therapy may adversely affect the community's general health.

With early advancements in well-researched illnesses and the possibility of new medicines, PM improves disease diagnosis and managed care. Genome sequencing is a valuable tool for identifying, monitoring, and managing outbreaks of infectious diseases. Newborn screening is also important for early detection of medical issues, which may help prevent complications and enhance infant health outcomes [11].

Genetics is essential in personalized medicine since it directs prevention, diagnosis, and therapy choices. Scientists are investigating uncommon or challenging medical conditions that lack treatments licensed by the FDA (Food and Drug Administration). AI is transforming healthcare by examining complex patterns in large datasets. Deep neural networks can forecast results and reveal concealed insights. Integrating AI with biomedical engineering enables more accurate diagnosis and tailored treatment approaches. This technology can identify illness biomarkers early, enhance treatment planning by considering an individual's genetics, lifestyle characteristics, and response patterns, and reduce side effects [12].

The remaining part of this chapter is organized as follows: Sec 2 delves into the background study of precision healthcare and elaborates on precision healthcare in Section 3. Section 4 provides the objectives of the proposed work, and challenges are discussed in Section 5. Section 6 discusses the applications and solutions of different techniques in precision healthcare. Section 7 elaborates on the discussion about precision healthcare applications and solutions. Section 8 gives the concluding remarks, followed by future work directions in precision healthcare.

BACKGROUND OF THE STUDY

The term "precision healthcare" refers to medical care that uses massive data sets of people, such as their genome or whole electronic health record, to customize the patient's medical treatment to their specific characteristics (shown in Fig. **2**). Precision healthcare is based on the idea that no two people are the same, and as a result, they should not get the same medical treatment. Precision Healthcare is a relatively new idea that focuses primarily on providing comprehensive treatment to patients. This will contribute to an increase in the availability of generic medications. A new strategy that utilizes information on an individual's genetic, environmental, and lifestyle information to guide choices relating to their medical treatment is known as precision healthcare [13]. This approach is comparable to personalized medicine or customized medicine.

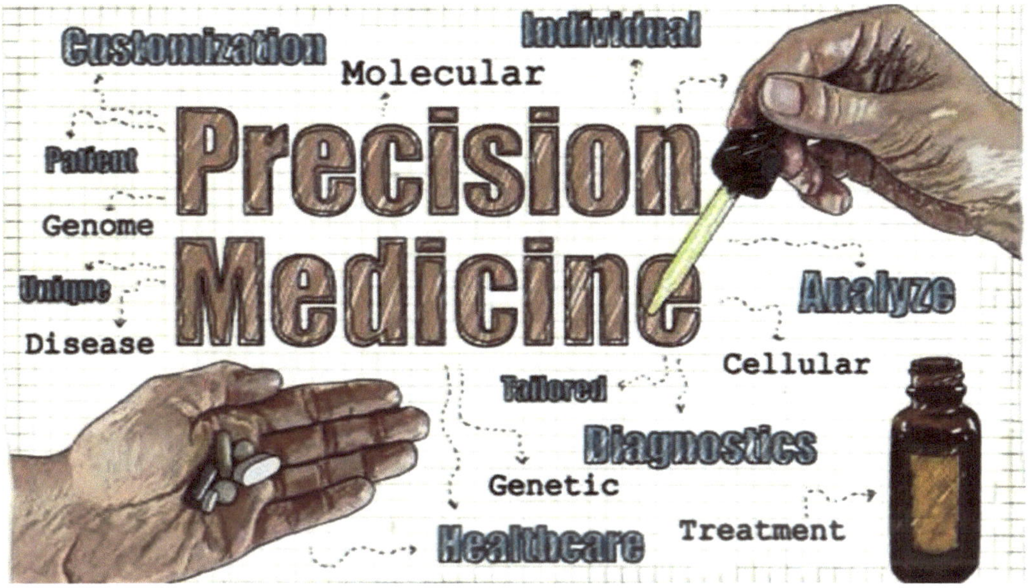

Fig. (2). The Role of Health Informatics in PM [14].

The notion of precision healthcare considers individual differences in genetics, environment, and lifestyle. Consequently, medical practitioners may select therapies most likely to benefit patients based on a more thorough understanding of the treated sickness or condition. Precision healthcare prioritizes the utilization of big data to deliver treatment that is both specific and individualized. In the healthcare sector, precision healthcare combines innovations from genomics, metabolomics, biomedical data sciences, and environmental sciences [15]. Numerous technical developments, such as mobile health, imaging, big data, artificial intelligence, social engagement, and networking, are utilized in this strategy. Precision healthcare refers to the convergence of individuals, their environment, alterations in diagnostic health indicators, and social and behavioral factors across time. Precision healthcare entails examining the elements that constitute individuals and populations and the dynamics of their changes and interactions across time. Even though the phrase "Precision Healthcare" has only been around for a short while, the idea behind it has been present in healthcare for quite some time [16]. For example, a person who requires a blood transfusion is not given blood from a donor chosen at random; instead, the donor's blood type is matched to the receiver to limit the likelihood of problems occurring after the transfusion.

Precision healthcare in biology, AI, digital health, and the move toward value-based care drive fast changes in healthcare and life science trends. The genomics market is expected to have a value of $38.7 billion by 2028 [17] because of the decreasing costs of DNA sequencing and the growing need for tailored therapy. AI and ML are revolutionizing drug development, diagnostics, and patient care. They enhance decision-making processes, allowing more efficient and precise tailored medicine [18].

The digital health industry is projected to reach $657.8 billion by 2026 [19], primarily due to the growing acceptance and use of telemedicine, remote patient monitoring, and mobile health technologies. These technologies allow patients to manage their health and enable healthcare practitioners to offer treatment that is easier to obtain, more efficient, and tailored to individual needs. Value-based care drives the need for novel healthcare delivery models that prioritize enhancing patient outcomes and decreasing costs.

RWD (Real-World Data) and RWE (Real-World Evidence) are transforming the healthcare and life sciences sector by supplying critical information for clinical decision-making, enabling the development of innovative therapies, and advancing the utilization of CDS (Clinical Decision Support) tools and SaMD (Software as a Medical Device) [20].

The growing comprehension of genetic, environmental, and lifestyle elements propels personalized medicine. Advancements in genomes, proteomics, and metabolomics facilitate the identification of novel biomarkers and treatment options. This leads to the development of personalized drugs and diagnostics specifically designed for an individual's unique characteristics [21].

ABOUT PRECISION HEALTHCARE

Precision healthcare entails the creation of precise methods that can effectively analyze individual data and its social context. These methods aim to extract concise descriptions with decreased complexity at the appropriate level of detail. These approaches must provide transparency, resilience, and flexibility in handling mistakes and uncertainty. Precision public health refers to the targeted delivery of appropriate interventions to specific populations at the optimal moment, which aligns with the often-mentioned concept of precision medicine. With backing from the Gates Foundation, Precision Public Health seeks to use data-driven ways to enhance overall population health and diminish health inequalities [22].

Precision public health focuses on tackling enduring socioeconomic conditions not addressed by clinical care, such as persistent social disparities in low-income nations. As it combines more data at the person level, precision public health is anticipated to need the scientific techniques associated with precision healthcare (shown in Fig. **3**). This approach will enable the incorporation of vaccination views, cultural context, unique medical records, DNA information, additional indicators, and personal danger signs into health care systems.

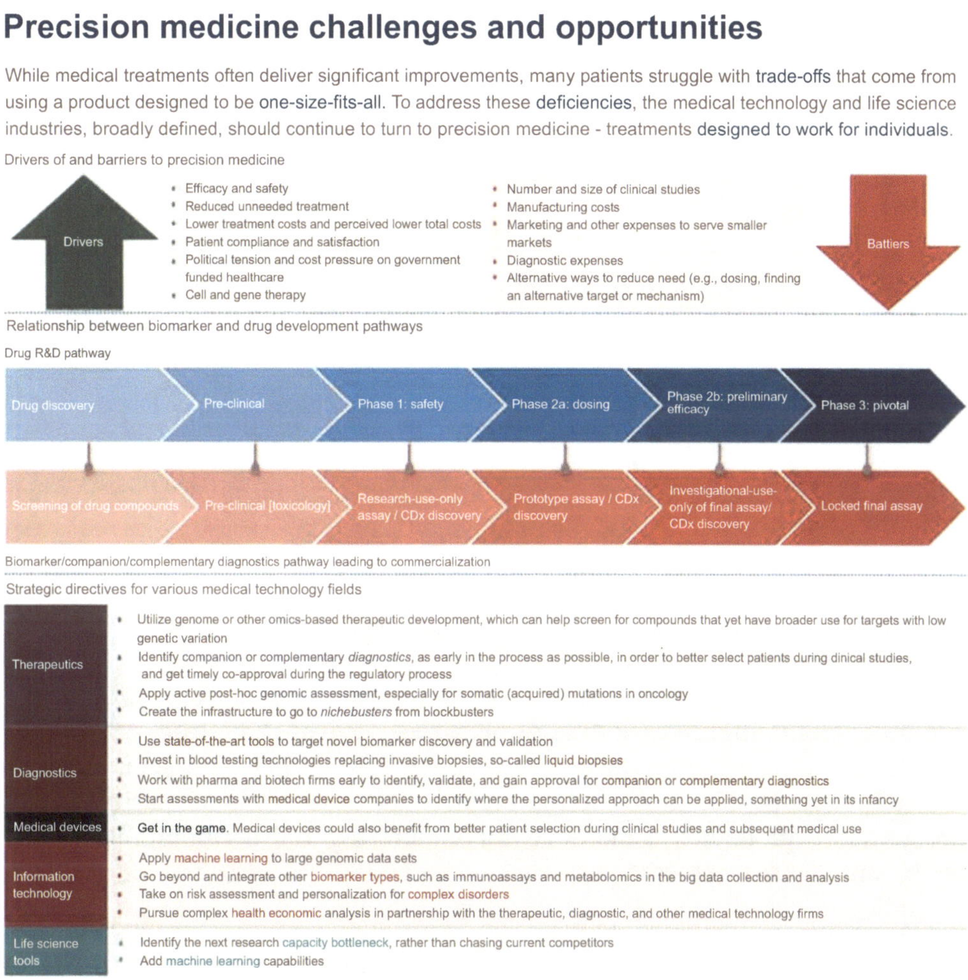

Fig. (3). Framework – PM challenges and opportunities [33].

The effectiveness of precision public health relies on addressing the mathematical obstacles identified in precision healthcare, including data analysis, stratification, modeling, using appropriate data to address specific inquiries, and preventing certain groups' unjust treatment *via* data misuse [23].

Customized therapies for groups with closely clustered biological traits have become the focal point of precision medicine, which was once known as individualized or customized medicine. Researchers have acknowledged that these routes may apply to a cohort of patients rather than individuals [24]. The objective is not to provide a distinct therapy for each individual or person, but to offer a more lucid comprehension of these cohorts.

EMRs (Electronic Medical Records)

EMRs are essential in PM since they provide a full perspective of a patient's health information, including medical history, diagnostic outcomes, and therapeutic interventions. This data may be used to create individualized therapeutic strategies customized to the patient's distinct genetic composition, surroundings, and way of life [25, 26]. Clinical decision support systems may enhance healthcare practitioners' treatment choices by examining this data. The rapid growth of EMR data clinical application, propelled by the HITECH Act [27], has resulted in an unparalleled surge of comprehensive, concentrated, and long-term clinical datasets. EMR data plays a vital role in the LHS Learning Healthcare System [28]. The LHS strives to effectively transform data on healthcare and operations into knowledge, which is then applied to evidence-based clinical practices and changes in the health system.

Nevertheless, there are difficulties associated with using EMR data for research and operations, mostly due to the heterogeneous and intricate structure of the data. Recent developments in informatics research have introduced alternative methods for automating the extraction and standardization of data. These methods include using NLP technologies to extract organized clinical data from unstructured narrative text and ontology-based techniques [29, 30]. Novel techniques and software platforms are now being created to bridge the disparity between unprocessed EMR data and the need for integrating and harmonizing Big Data based on ontological concepts [31].

Drug Discovery

This is an ever-expanding subject that includes cutting-edge approaches like gene therapy and immunotherapies. Nevertheless, scientists encounter a multitude of obstacles, including escalating expenses, constraints in modeling, and misconstrued illness processes. To enhance research outcomes, the industry needs to decrease expenses and improve the efficiency of discoveries. With the progress of research in new modeling technologies, it is essential to evaluate the existing endeavors and ascertain their effectiveness in addressing these difficulties [32].

The success rate of drug development projects is very low, with just 4% leading to the licensing of medicines and biologics, and less than 10% achieving success in clinical trials. The primary reason for failure is a deficiency in providing clear evidence of effectiveness, which arises from initial mistakes made while identifying or validating the target. Preclinical research conducted in cells, tissues, and animal models is not a replica of human diseases, and using limited sample numbers might result in inaccurate positive findings. AI and ML techniques can quickly and accurately discover new chemicals and targets. Additionally, receiving feedback on unfavorable outcomes may improve the accuracy of future prediction models. Using data in drug research is anticipated to enhance drug development initiatives by reducing costs and fostering creativity [33]. However, certain prerequisites need to be fulfilled: 1) the data must be impartial, 2) it should include various forms of data, and 3) a willingness to share the data. Utilizing genomics to find drugs, based on Genome-Wide Association Studies (GWAS), has the potential to simplify the process. However, the limited variety in many GWAS cohorts may result in false illness connections [34].

The pandemic caused by COVID-19 has brought to light the significance of AI, ML, and Deep Learning (DL) technologies in developing medications and vaccines. These technologies accelerate the process, minimizing labor-intensive, costly, and time-consuming procedures. Pharmaceutical businesses are progressively using AI technologies such as Deep Learning for medication creation and testing. These techniques need thorough data analysis because of the many chemical combinations involved. AI systems can efficiently process and analyze enormous amounts of data, resulting in accelerated medication development, speedier market release, and reduced costs [35].

Effective management of precision oncology data requires strong data governance to safeguard patient confidentiality and facilitate open sharing for clinical and research objectives. Nevertheless, patients often voice apprehensions over the possible misapplication of their data [36], which might result in exploitation and prejudice. Currently, there is a lack of complete global legislation on data privacy. To avert re-identification, it is recommended that comprehensive systems, including access control, data anonymization, and encryption, be employed [37]. Patients want a more precise comprehension of the utilization and objectives of data, and there is a necessity for public standards to ensure that data is employed and disseminated safely and openly [38]. Blockchain technology is being praised as a viable method to tackle the complexities of data exchange while safeguarding patient privacy. Patients are empowered to make decisions regarding their involvement in research and using their data for research purposes by deploying prototype platforms created by the Australian Genomics Health Alliance. Enhancing the framework of the medical system is necessary to ensure information regarding patient sovereignty. This requires the development of a solid digital infrastructure as well as an evaluation of the effectiveness of either centralized or decentralized data storage. Patients must have a comprehensive comprehension of genetic data and an awareness of the methods often used in clinical genomics [39].

The ability to store, integrate, and analyze data depends on on-premises technologies for firms in the healthcare industry. On the other hand, these methods often fail to meet the requirements of the extensive and complex datasets used in precision oncology. It is estimated that around eighty percent of medical data is kept in an unstructured format, necessitating complex techniques such as NLP or human analysis. Even though there have been advancements in data abstraction, there are concerns about the scalability of NLP in standard care settings because it is not cost-effective. Many resources are required to address the problem of missing and inconsistent data, which may not be proportionate to the therapeutic advantages obtained [40, 41]. It is vital to organize and efficiently prepare data to achieve a level of quality in healthcare that is both cost-effective and efficient. The objective of the project known as the mCODE (minimal Common Oncology Data Elements) is to provide a basic definition of data to address the problem of data standardization in the field of cancer [42]. A framework to enhance healthcare data interoperability has been established by the Global Alliance for Genomics and Health, since the absence of interoperability hinders data interchange. The principal challenges regarding data sharing are primarily associated with financial limits, with the cost component being a significant barrier to the broad application of the practice. However, several nation and region-specific projects have recognized the benefits of sharing data, which has helped to avoid the need for a compulsory centralized data storage system [43].

Emergency care settings [44] have limited decision-making time and a little margin for mistakes. Therefore, integrating PM technology with Clinical Medicine is very helpful in high-pressure circumstances. A patient having trouble breathing, known as dyspnea, may be assessed and prioritized using a biomarker score, such as the Manchester Triage Score. If there is a pressing need to determine the source of a condition, and considering the clinical, epidemiologic, and sociodemographic factors, it would be advisable to use a diagnostic biomarker panel to distinguish between distinct causes. The mentioned biomarkers include high-sensitivity cardiac troponin T, d-Dimer, brain natriuretic peptide, C-reactive Protein (CRP), procalcitonin, and pro-adrenomedullin. High sensitivity T is indicative of cardiac injury, d-Dimer is used to rule out venous thromboembolism, brain natriuretic peptide is an indicator of heart failure, C-reactive Protein (CRP) is used to guide response to therapy in cases of infection and inflammation, procalcitonin prompts the use of microbiological cultures and antimicrobial treatment, and pro-adrenomedullin is a newer biomarker that has a superior prognosis value compared to C-reactive Protein (CRP) and ProCalciTonin (PCT). This method is especially beneficial in cases of community-acquired pneumonia and other diseases affecting the respiratory system.

Genomic and transcriptome analyses have shown encouraging findings in detecting vasculopathy alterations linked to the APOE allele in acute care environments. These investigations have provided valuable insights for guiding treatment and care decisions, identifying Single Nucleotide Polymorphisms (SNPs) linked to stroke recanalization, and distinguishing between individuals with ischemic and non-ischaemic cardiomyopathy. Biomarkers such as CRP, IL-6, and procalcitonin have been used to forecast unfavourable results in COVID-19, distinguish sepsis from SIRS, and anticipate severe sepsis and septic shock. The discovery of these results has sparked the development of emergency precision medicine. This framework encompasses an electronic health record system, previous medical visits, fundamental patient information, research advancements, and primary care screening data. This technique facilitates intricate decision-making in acute situations, providing clinicians and patients with enhanced medical treatment.

Precision Healthcare and Life Science

Precision health integrates preventive measures and wellness practices with disease management. However, no one entity has the necessary resources, solutions, expertise, and data to adequately address the comprehensive healthcare requirements of individuals throughout their whole lives. A precision health system requires an ecosystem approach encompassing several stakeholders, such as healthcare providers, payers, pharmaceutical companies, tech businesses, employers, governments, and social groups. The transition to precision health can enhance human well-being and provide substantial cost savings by preventing diseases, facilitating early intervention, avoiding incorrect diagnoses and treatments, and refining medication and diagnostic research and development. An advanced precision health system (shown in Fig. **4**) would provide comprehensive guidance for patients' health and well-being, using genetic predisposition, risk factors, biomarkers, preventive interventions, and frequent monitoring [45].

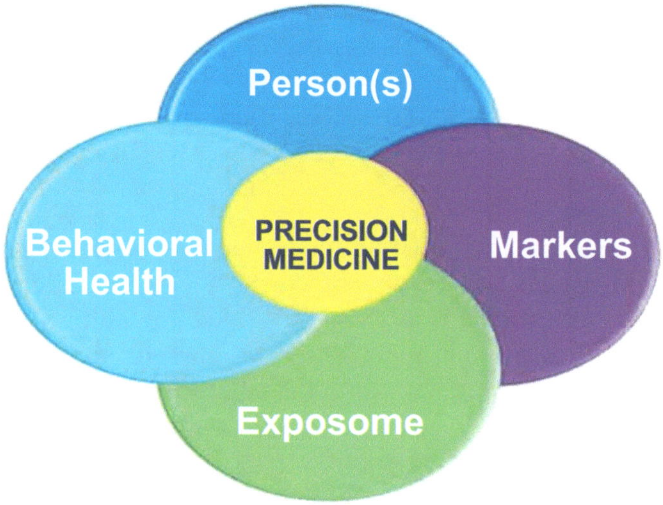

Fig. (4). The person(s), markers, exposome, and behavioral health are the components of the PM paradigm, which is shown by a Venn diagram [46].

OBJECTIVES OF PRECISION HEALTHCARE

Person(s): For healthcare practitioners to better manage population health, detect and resolve healthcare inequities, and improve patient care, patient demographics are essential. The personal information included in this category comprises age, gender, race, ethnicity, marital status, education, employment, insurance, and contact details. Healthcare professionals gather this data by asking unambiguous questions, ensuring privacy and confidentiality, and using brief language. Examining patient demographic data may provide valuable insights for enhancing community health management and patient care. Approaches to tackling healthcare inequalities include comprehending gaps, delivering culturally proficient treatment, enhancing healthcare accessibility, diminishing financial obstacles, and using demographics in healthcare planning [47].

Markers: An interdisciplinary strategy founded on six scientific pillars is known as precision health. The genomic medicine pillar focuses on studying the genetic elements that impact the development of diseases and the effectiveness of treatment interventions. The pillar of cell, gene, and immune treatment focuses on investigating immune response mechanisms and developing therapies. Chemical biology and biotherapeutics primarily study the biological processes influenced by gene expression or protein function. Data and informatics play a vital role in the analysis and storage of data. The behavioral, psychological, and ethical pillars guarantee ethical research and healthcare practice. Regenerative medicine and engineering aim to generate functioning tissues to replace lost tissue or organ function [48].

Exposome: The exposome is a theoretical framework that quantifies an individual's cumulative exposures during their lifespan and examines how these exposures, which include environmental and occupational factors, interact with genetics, physiology, and epigenetics to impact health. Exposomics is the scientific field that investigates the exposome using several evaluation techniques, both internal and external. These techniques include genomics, metabonomics, lipidomics, transcriptomics, and proteomics. The exposome has the potential to significantly transform our understanding of illness etiology and contribute to the development of preventive measures and treatments for a wider range of disorders. Genetics, while influential, only contributes to 10% of illnesses, whereas the other reasons are ascribed to environmental factors. The progress of exposomics encounters obstacles such as the considerable variability in an individual's exposome, the influence of exposures that change throughout different phases of life, and the difficulties of comprehensively mapping the whole of an exposome due to its intricate structure [49].

Behavioral Health: Biology, emotions, and behaviors that are connected to mental health are studied in behavioral health. Precision health seeks to enhance therapies by providing tailored assistance by integrating genetic or genomic data with contextual information. The evaluation was conducted using clinical assessment, individualized treatment, and digital health using computer algorithms and automated procedures [50]. Health-monitoring gadgets and sophisticated algorithms are preferred owing to their scalability and cost-effectiveness, making them perfect for a hands-off approach. Nevertheless, human-led, low-tech customization may hinder the ability to efficiently expand behavior modification interventions at a reasonable cost [51]. Additional research is required in Randomized Controlled Trials (RCTs) and health economic evaluations to optimize the effectiveness and cost-effectiveness of interventions. The precision healthcare paradigm, as suggested by [52], showcases the potential of digital technology in gathering data, monitoring health conditions, assessing risks, and analyzing data. Upcoming therapies may use wearable devices for streamlined data collection and monitoring, as well as ML and predictive modeling for improved data analysis and risk evaluation.

Optimal treatment: PM is a medical methodology that comprehensively comprehends an individual's traits and symptoms to discern appropriate therapies and preventive measures. It enhances results, minimizes negative consequences, enhances patient involvement, and decreases expenses. Columbia University Medical Center- New York Presbyterian employs genetics and information technology to make well-informed judgments, systematically categorizing the risk of diseases and discovering the most effective means of care. This method offers more precise prognostic data, allowing for tailored treatments with greater success rates, reduced risk of negative responses, improved cost-effectiveness, and enhanced patient outcomes [53].

Detect genetic alterations associated with diseases: PM is a medical approach that focuses on treating illnesses by targeting specific gene abnormalities and changing the precise genes involved to cure patients. It became popular with the introduction of the PM—initiative by Barack Obama, which focuses explicitly on cancer and diabetes. The program seeks to combat illnesses using a tailored strategy, specifically targeting and rectifying faulty genes by direct eradication, restoration, correction, or repair. Nevertheless, the incorporation of genetic testing into personalized cancer treatments and decision-making continues to present difficulties. PM is an extension of clinical and translational medicine that offers a novel option for established therapy. It can potentially significantly affect disease cures and patient prognoses [54].

Using predictive biomarkers, personalized medicine maximizes patient outcomes by using genetic profiles. Pharmacogenomics, which investigates the relationship between genes and drugs, is crucial in developing biomarkers in other "omics" disciplines. Scientists are investigating uncommon or challenging medical conditions and those that do not have treatments authorized by the FDA, while the field of cancer is seeing tremendous growth as a therapeutic area [55].

Minimize the occurrence of severe adverse reactions caused by drugs: The use of PM reduces treatment toxicity and damage to healthy cells by tailoring medicines to genetic aberrations in cancer. Genetic testing and screening facilitate the early identification and diagnosis of diseases, allowing for timely interventions. Additionally, it enhances clinical trials by specifically targeting genetic anomalies and identifying patient subgroups for innovative treatments.

CHALLENGES OF PRECISION HEALTHCARE

Ensuring the prevention of diseases is of utmost importance for promoting good health and well-being among the population. However, Under Represented Minority (URM) communities in the United States are particularly vulnerable to higher risks and poorer health outcomes. This is primarily due to factors such as a lack of trust in the healthcare system, limited access to healthcare facilities due to geographical distance, language barriers, and concerns about encountering implicit bias and stereotyping during medical care. Conventional medical methods may provide inconsistent outcomes because they do not include the fundamental social, cultural, environmental, and lifestyle elements influencing health [56]. Conventional medical procedures may also result in a limited presence of Under Represented Minority (URM) individuals in genetic registries and clinical trials, resulting in an uneven distribution of treatment choices. These populations are less likely to obtain treatments due to the direct implications of precision medicine, which typically uses genetic data for patient treatment regimens. Genome-wide Association Studies (GWAS) seldom examine the correlation between intricate genetic characteristics and environmental exposure [57]. The field of PM shows potential to improve health outcomes, especially for urban and rural populations that have limited access to medical care. Nevertheless, a typical issue emerges from the absence of precise demographic classifications, which leads to uneven misrepresentation or characterization of underrepresented populations in clinical trials [58].

Addressing the problematic interaction between Under Represented Minority (URM) and clinical trials is crucial since long-term research projects sometimes continue to have unfavorable associations long beyond their original intention [59].

The incorporation of precision healthcare into everyday clinical treatment has significant challenges, including a lack of available tools, a restricted knowledge base, and research gaps.

Requirements for Infrastructure

Precision healthcare has the potential to influence healthcare significantly, but to do this, it requires significant expenditures in infrastructure [54] and a significant amount of time to deploy. To implement precision healthcare, it is necessary to make significant modifications to the infrastructure and the method for collecting, storing, and exchanging data.

Constitutional Challenges

A significant amount of genetic data must be gathered from a vast and varied cross-section of the population for Precision Healthcare to achieve its full potential in terms of efficiency. In situations when such an enormous volume of data is gathered, it is difficult to determine who the legal owner of the data is.

Opportunities

One of the most significant developments in precision healthcare is the use of technologies such as AI, the IoT, and big data to develop new healthcare delivery models [60]. Algorithms from AI and ML can examine enormous datasets, therefore recognizing patterns and connections that medical professionals may miss. In the meantime, IoT devices provide real-time monitoring and data collection, which results in a more complete information profile of the patient. Even though this convergence of technology and healthcare creates enormous prospects for customized therapy, it also brings problems, such as the need for advanced analytic tools and concerns over data privacy. The research underscores this paradigm shift and emphasizes the significance of harnessing AI and ML algorithms to assess enormous information produced by "omics" technologies5 for the benefit of physicians and patients in real-time. This request intends to stimulate the development of technologies and methods that bring personalized medicine closer to reality, ultimately providing more accurate, predictive, and preventative healthcare solutions. This will be accomplished by stressing the role that AI [61] plays in unlocking the value of multi-omic and clinical data.

To develop and verify new biomarkers and responses to therapy, phenotyping technologies [62] make it possible to get a more profound knowledge of human physiology and illness with a specificity that has never been seen before. High-throughput omics technologies, such as transcriptomics, proteomics, metabolomics, microbiome profiling, flow cytometry, and electronic biomarkers, such as actigraphy (the assessment of patient movement in real-time using mobile sensors), are some of these technologies.

Technological Challenges

Overfitting and Underfitting

ML applications in healthcare provide potential advantages as well as difficulties. The risks include potential inaccuracies in predictions, susceptibility of the system to attacks, concerns over protecting personal information, and challenges related to data availability. Furthermore, there are notable ethical considerations, decreased human interaction, and challenges related to interpretability. Probabilistic distribution gives rise to doubt over the accuracy of forecasts. Machine learning-based techniques may lead to a significant loss of human life. To reduce these dangers, it is necessary to get strong institutional and legal permission [63]. Medical experts' involvement may prevent inaccurate diagnoses, whether false-positive or false-negative. Engaging healthcare workers in the development of ML may enhance the pace of adoption and alleviate worries about workforce reduction [64].

Interpretability and Explainability

Interpretability and explainability: Transparency and ethical issues are key to the dependability of AI-based medical equipment, and comprehension of the outcomes is essential. Regulations impose more stringent criteria for evaluating the explainability and interpretability of AI-based device selections, guaranteeing that stakeholders are held accountable [65]. AI systems should provide physicians and patients with a thorough comprehension of terminal illnesses, with a focus on emphasizing the capacity to explain in the healthcare field. It is possible to select high explainability models by employing explainable AI techniques such as Local Interpretable Model-agnostic Explanations, Anchors, Graph Local Interpretable Model Explanations, Shapley Flow, Textual Explanations of Visual Models [66], Integrated Gradients, Causal Models, and Meaningful Perturbations [67].

Several factors undermine the trustworthiness of AI-based medical informatics, including the scarcity of randomized clinical trials, a lack of transparency, the possibility of biases, and ambiguous laws [68].

Observational Data and Causality

Causality is a fundamental notion used in observational research to examine how a system might react to an intervention. It aids in determining cause-and-effect relationships and measuring their extent concerning risk variables and their influence on health and social consequences. It is necessary to ascertain the potential impacts of exposure and non-exposure on an individual to establish causality between a particular exposure and a result. Nevertheless, it is challenging to establish definitive causal effects for individual cases using observational data, as we can only witness the result for a particular person under a single potential exposure value [69]. Inferring population causal effects from observed relationships between variables may be challenging when dealing with missing data since it involves making assumptions that cannot be tested due to confounding, selection, and measurement issues [70]. The use of observational data to deduce causal treatment effects has gained popularity in recent years, mainly owing to advancements in EHRs and ML methodologies [71, 72].

Algorithmic Bias

AI technology provides many advantages, but it also poses ethical and legal difficulties, such as bias in trained algorithms, the need for diverse data representation, and the preservation of patient privacy. Utilizing AI is of utmost importance for physicians and researchers, with the caveat of ensuring impartiality and accurately reflecting the worldwide population. AI systems need input data for training and discerning patterns, and the precision of predictions is contingent upon this data. Significant concerns also include racial prejudice, sex-specific bias, patient risk assessments, cost-quality of treatment, and therapeutic responses. To tackle these problems, healthcare data scientists and developers should use effective strategies such as involving various individuals to evaluate and oversee algorithms and AI systems, handling instances when there is inadequate information, collaborating with multiple groups, and establishing mechanisms for receiving input [73].

Validation and Generalizability

Thorough and methodical validation of AI technologies is essential for their incorporation into clinical practice to avoid unintended damage, such as incorrect diagnosis, unsuitable therapy, or adverse consequences, which might reduce patient survival rates. Only a limited number of AI-based systems have undergone clinical validation, mostly using internal datasets, without external validation. Retrospective Clinical Trials (RCTs) are the most robust and dependable method for evaluating the performance and safety of AI [74]. However, they are expensive and should be preceded by preliminary investigations. Once AI technologies reach a state of full development, they must undergo clinical validation using external real-world datasets. This process enables the efficient and dependable assessment of AI performance and safety in real-life circumstances. If an AI fails to meet expectations, it might be dismissed without the need for any further review. Validation should be essential to the overall AI assessment process [75].

Incorporating Multimorbidity

Multimorbidity, which refers to many pre-existing comorbidities, is becoming an increasingly worrisome issue within the healthcare system. It affects more than 60% of individuals in the US who are 65 years or older and is especially common in critical care settings. Patients with hypertension, diabetes mellitus, and chronic obstructive pulmonary disease often experience higher expenses, negative events, and poorer results compared to those without additional health conditions [76, 77]. Recovery from critical illness might also be affected by pre-existing chronic disease. Nevertheless, our comprehension of multi-morbid people is often flawed, since some individuals are disregarded based on criteria such as "underlying disease with unfavorable prognosis." The presence and measurability of multimorbidity [78] may hinder the development of precision critical care, as it may not be tied to distinct clusters that inform treatment decisions. It may also be included in the collection of factors assessed while determining distinct groupings. Investigating multimorbidity as a causative factor in phenotypic variation might include examining its potential impact on the epigenome [79]. Twin concordance studies provide evidence for the role of epigenetics in illness since they reveal that heritable characteristics associated with different types of cancer are present in a varying percentage of twin pairs [80].

Economic Relevance

PM is an intricate discipline that encompasses customized therapies informed by genetic, environmental, and lifestyle variables. The complicated nature of the subject makes it challenging to apply generalizations on costs and results to various patient demographics. The implementation and use of precision medicine, which encompasses genetic testing and individualized medication creation, might incur significant expenses, prompting inquiries over cost-effectiveness. The trade-off between long-term advantages and current expenses is a substantial obstacle in precision medicine. This is because PM significantly depends on the gathering and analysis of data, which in turn raises issues over patient confidentiality and the security of data. Implementing novel therapies faces obstacles in terms of payment and regulatory matters. Insurance companies and healthcare providers are grappling with creating frameworks to support these treatments.

Additionally, measuring outcomes is difficult owing to the personalized nature of the treatments. Equity and access concerns provide an additional obstacle, since PM may only be accessible to those who possess the financial means or reside in sophisticated healthcare systems [81]. Tackling these obstacles may facilitate the development of more economically efficient therapies in the future, resulting in more engagement in clinical trials and perhaps expanding the accessibility of efficacious medications in the market.

Governance

A strong data governance foundation is essential to modernizing healthcare, with an emphasis on data standards to boost interoperability. Interoperability guarantees smooth and uninterrupted access to data across different systems, devices, and applications, maximizing health outcomes. Data governance is a process that establishes the management of crucial data assets, guaranteeing Trust and responsibility for adverse events caused by poor data quality. Health systems may exchange data by adhering to established standards such as Health Level-7, clinical and message format standards, Digital Imaging and Communications in Medicine (DICOM), International Classification of Diseases, Tenth Revision (ICD-10), and Fast Healthcare Interoperability Resources (FHIR). However, data governance challenges develop when both parties lack communication or understanding, necessitating a translator to get relevant insights. Data governance enhances the process of analyzing, doing analytics, comprehending, conducting in-depth searches, and gaining insights from data [82]. This has a significant influence on clinical decision-making and drives efforts related to population health.

The data must possess accuracy, accessibility, comprehensiveness, consistency, currency, clear definition, and relevance to the objective of the patient interaction. The content should be devoid of mistakes, accurate, and current. It is essential to establish appropriate measures to guarantee the accessibility of data. The data must be complete, consistent, and up-to-date, with all aspects precisely specified and at a suitable degree of detail. The data should be both current and accurate [83].

Scalability and Generalization

The capacity of a technology solution to be scaled up is an essential component to consider when determining its efficacy. In the healthcare industry, the term "scalability" refers to the capacity of a system, network, or process to handle an increasing quantity of work or to expand to accommodate additional work. This might suggest that physicians are responsible for a greater number of patients, managing an expanded amount of data, or integrating more complicated processes.

Generalization in cognitive science enables the identification of commonalities in acquired information from one context, enabling the application of that knowledge to other scenarios. In predictive modeling in clinical activities, generalizability refers to a model's ability to effectively perform its intended function using data from a separate group of patients, like external validation. Suppose a model fails to meet this description. In that case, it may not have accurately learned the link between characteristics and the intended result, or may have acquired biases from data generation and processing. Around 23% of machine learning-based healthcare articles use more than one dataset, making it difficult to generalize findings across different centers. Validating a model using just one dataset, even if it is from the same group of individuals as the training data, is not recommended. To enhance the availability of ML healthcare models in various hospital environments, different methods of customizing models are necessary to adapt them to sites and facilitate their implementation in new settings [84].

Ethical Considerations

PM is a hopeful strategy for treating and preventing diseases, but it may worsen health inequalities if it fails to include environmental influences. The issues it poses include obtaining informed permission, disclosing genetic risks within families, and dealing with prejudice. Personalizing health hazards heightens the likelihood of people being held accountable for their health problems. The information foundation for PM is derived from genetic research, which mainly includes individuals of European origin, hence restricting equitable advantages for other populations. The exorbitant expense of PM therapies generates apprehensions about the accessibility and equitable allocation of prospective advantages, especially for uncommon ailments or precision [85].

Interdisciplinary Collaboration

Interdisciplinary collaboration entails the cooperative efforts of specialists from several fields to provide exceptional care to patients, caregivers, and communities. Precision medicine exemplifies this integrative approach.

Precision medicine, an extensively used subject in medical domains such as internal medicine, surgery, and cancer, depends on fundamental technologies from several disciplines, such as genomics technology, big data, and nanobiotechnology. Nevertheless, the advancement of PM encounters several obstacles and necessitates substantial multidisciplinary collaboration. PM is an interdisciplinary discipline with several topic categories, as shown by the assignment of subject categories by the Web of Science [86].

Interdisciplinary cooperation entails integrating information from several disciplines to establish new study domains. Historically, it has served as an indicator of the progress and advancements in research. Researchers in clinical and translational science need tools to find resources and work together. Researchers in information behavior and library sciences have investigated multidisciplinary cooperation using bibliometrics and co-word analysis techniques to gain insights into its characteristics.

Explainability and Trust

Explainability, also known as interpretability, refers to the capacity of an ML model to be comprehensible to a person. Explainable AI (XAI) is essential in the healthcare field because it improves the transparency and interpretability of decision-making processes powered by AI. Integrating XAI with PM can enhance treatment results for many illnesses by offering understandable and meaningful insights from intricate multi-modal data. Additionally, XAI technologies may enhance the quality of patient care by improving patient expectations, perception, and experience, ultimately resulting in optimal treatment results. Collaboration across different disciplines is crucial for making progress in XAI in the healthcare field and building confidence among healthcare providers and patients. Trust is essential in the healthcare field due to the presence of ambiguity and potential risks for vulnerable patients who depend on the expertise and intentions of healthcare professionals. Trust is the unwavering confidence in an individual or entity's dependability, veracity, or competence [87, 88].

Better care, more treatment acceptance and adherence, less anxiety, and simpler access to health services correlate with Trust in healthcare providers. Patients are more inclined to provide information, and the level of communication increases, leading to increased patient independence and collaborative decision-making. Confidence in healthcare workers also improves patient engagement.

Patient Empowerment and Education

PM is an innovative methodology that collects and analyzes extensive data on a patient's medical history, lifestyle, genetic makeup, and environmental influences to customize the optimal therapy for the patient. Patient empowerment is the systematic acquisition of increased authority and influence over choices and behaviors that impact one's well-being.

Empower the Patient with Knowledge and Skills

Psycho Education

Schedule sessions with a therapist or counsellor to understand the nature of the anxiety disorder, triggers, and coping mechanisms.

Skill Development

Train the patient in relaxation techniques like deep breathing, mindfulness exercises, and progressive muscle relaxation.

Educational Resources

Provide access to websites, self-help books, and apps with information on anxiety management and self-care.

Socioeconomic Impacts

Socioeconomic effects are the consequences of a community's self-identification, cultural practices, traditions, language, demographic attributes, and economic foundation on its primary industries, employment trends, and infrastructure. Socioeconomic factors such as income, employment, housing, and education may impact an individual's health. Disadvantaged persons may have challenges obtaining healthcare, which can, therefore, influence their general health and well-being.

APPLICATIONS AND SOLUTIONS FOR PRECISION HEALTHCARE

Precision health apps use a variety of data sources to evaluate potential hazards, make diagnoses, and implement proactive therapies. These metrics include biological, genetic, environmental, social, and lifestyle factors. Although clinical and community-based health data sources are not yet completely established, it is feasible to integrate PM and Social Determinants of Health (SDOH) into the same therapies. This strategy entails the establishment of dynamic connections between medicine, economics, population health, and public health [89].

Healthcare firms deal with constant issues due to a lack of data, technology, and insight. To tackle these problems, it is essential to prioritize modernization and data governance. AI may be used to apply sophisticated knowledge to data, boost the availability of patients' comprehensive health records, and optimize workflow, analysis, and cooperation across care teams. These actions will substantially affect patient treatment and the management of an aging population. Equipping organizations to provide individualized medicine will enhance results and align with the concepts of value-based care. Advancing technology is crucial for ensuring the delivery of state-of-the-art, high-quality healthcare to all individuals.

Precision Healthcare employs innovative technology and methodologies to categorize and ascertain the origins of different diseases to treat and prevent them. Precision Healthcare [90] utilizes several tools such as molecular diagnostics, imaging, and analytics. Precision healthcare and personalized medicine, also known as customized medicine, include using an individual's genetic profile to inform clinical choices on illness prevention, diagnosis, and treatment. The empirical algorithm for Precision Healthcare aims to find medications and pharmacological targets *via* testing.

- Develop a disease model with high accuracy that accurately portrays a patient's specific illness.
- Characterize the illness model with accuracy.
- Evaluate candidate treatments using the illness concept.

If no prospective treatments are found, trials will be conducted to identify drug targets. Afterward, these drug targets will be input into the high-level algorithm for Precision Healthcare to discover potential therapeutics.

Apply the possible treatments revealed by the model to human subjects.

Precision Healthcare [91] has great promise for revolutionizing the healthcare industry by enhancing treatment results, minimizing unwanted effects, and decreasing healthcare expenses.

Benefits

The emphasis in medicine should be redirected towards prevention rather than reaction. This involves giving priority to predicting one's vulnerability to diseases, improving the detection of diseases, preventing the progression of diseases, customizing strategies for disease prevention, prescribing more effective drugs, avoiding predictable side effects, minimizing the duration, expenses, and inability percentage of clinical studies, and removing ineffectiveness linked to trial-an--error methods. Additionally, it is crucial to consider the applications of genetic diseases and evaluate the risk of genetic cancer [92].

Although there are still obstacles to overcome, the potential advantages of customized medicine [93] in improving patient care and decreasing healthcare expenses are significant. With ongoing advancements in understanding the human genome and using data analytics, Precision Healthcare is ready to revolutionize the healthcare field. AI in Precision Healthcare [94] has completely transformed how healthcare is provided. Precision Healthcare characterizes the phenotype of specific individuals who exhibit uncommon reactions to therapy. Recent studies have shown that translational research on the intersection of AI and Precision Healthcare will aid in resolving the most complex issues in Precision Healthcare. In this discussion, we explore many facets of AI in Precision Healthcare that enhance the delivery of healthcare services. "P4 Medicine" refers to a clinical medicine model based on four key principles: Predictive, Preventive, Personalized, and Participative. This model offers tangible opportunities to change the healthcare paradigm. The active involvement of the individual is crucial in implementing the other three aspects of P4 with each patient.

Although significant improvements have been made in information systems, computer science, and mathematics, developing and using ML models continues to be difficult. The data is partitioned into two sets: the training and testing sets. The training set is used to educate the model, while the model's performance is assessed based on its description of the testing set. Nevertheless, real-world data is seldom random and might exhibit temporal patterns that can influence the accuracy of predictions [95].

PM necessitates efficiently extracting complex data from several domains, including clinical, biological, patient-generated, and environmental. AI, specifically ML, plays a crucial role in facilitating this. ML has already been effectively used to automate mundane clinical procedures, such as prioritizing patient orders in the emergency room or assessing medical images. The combination of increased computer power, data availability, advanced algorithms, and increased interest from healthcare researchers has led to a significant increase in rigorous studies focused on discovering and implementing precision medicine. Nevertheless, to guarantee the practicality and effectiveness of the clinical application, it is essential to address the methodological obstacles and provide a comprehensive framework that produces compelling proof of patient safety and benefits while meeting all regulatory standards [96].

The widespread implementation of precision oncology is impeded by significant limitations associated with funding and reimbursement. Suggested approaches for effectively implementing public-private finance agreements and performance-based payment systems have been proposed [97]. Nevertheless, obstacles emerge because of the lack of connection between the educational and commercial fields, discrepancies in research objectives, ethical and legal issues concerning the sharing of data and samples, the production of result data, and the challenge of implementing risk-sharing agreements across different healthcare systems. The existing health technology assessment frameworks do not address the uncertainties linked to precision oncology medicines [98]. Create a comprehensive strategy with pragmatic recommendations for adequate finance and payment solutions for PM in diverse healthcare systems throughout Europe. The primary recommendations entail augmenting public and philanthropic funding in research and development, establishing global study organizations and collaborative spaces to facilitate the sharing of public-private research, implementing a legal framework, establishing comprehensive pan-European databases, leveraging funding arrangements, and improving openness concerning cost and refund. These recommendations aim to guide medical organizations in developing strategic policy measures to provide affordable and efficient access to PM standards of care for all.

PM is an essential component of healthcare that emphasizes tailored and efficient therapy for disorders. The Obama administration initiated the Precision Medicine Initiative (PMI) in the United States, intending to examine the genetic origins of illnesses. Similarly, the UK government intends to provide 210 million towards advancing cutting-edge diagnostic technologies, medicinal goods, and therapies rooted in precision medicine. The National Academy of Medicine (NAM) prioritizes the quality of treatment in areas such as efficacy, efficiency, well-being, justice, patient-centeredness, and timeliness [99]. Deep Learning (DL) models are very effective analytical tools in healthcare because they can accurately represent many kinds of data, such as text, pictures, videos, audio, and other complicated data formats [100]. Convolutional neural networks, recurrent neural networks, and deep belief networks are advanced computational models that can handle large and diverse datasets. These models can uncover fascinating patterns that cannot be discovered with shallow learning methods [101]. Incorporating omics data has significantly influenced functional genomics, with a wide range of applications including patient care, medication development, and discovery [102]. This study intends to analyze PM utilizing Deep Learning models and explore its potential by offering multidisciplinary research that supports precision medicine-based healthcare services.

ML algorithms examine integrated information to find patterns, correlations, and prediction linkages. Convolutional Neural Networks (CNNs) and advanced Deep Learning architectures are trained using labeled datasets to accurately identify complex patterns in biological data. Transfer learning approaches improve the ability of a model to generalize by using knowledge gained from one dataset to enhance the analysis of many medical scenarios. These AI models serve as the foundation for individualized diagnoses and treatment planning, precisely forecasting the risk and course of diseases, and enabling early intervention and preventative actions [103].

Data science methodologies are essential for categorizing risk and preventing diseases, using genetic, epigenomic, exposomic, proteomic, and metabolomic data. Artificial intelligence, including ML and NLP, can detect patterns in intricate datasets, such as environmental exposure measures. Using this information, AI may accurately identify people or communities susceptible to negative consequences. High-dimensional data analysis is enhanced by precision environmental health, which necessitates using rigorous data science methods to comprehend the effects of environmental exposures and create risk stratification [104]. By using many types of biological data in precision environmental health research [105], we may better understand how exposures affect health. This approach goes beyond studying observable characteristics and focuses on the underlying genetic and molecular factors. We may develop focused therapies and achieve precise disease prevention by integrating mechanistic knowledge of how exposures contribute to illness, the accompanying biological responses, and the omic-based factors that determine disease risk.

SECURITY, PRIVACY, AND RELIABILITY OF HEALTH CARE DATA

Precision medical data protection uses Anonymization and de-identification procedures to preserve patient privacy. Adhering to privacy standards such as HIPAA is essential for researchers and healthcare organizations to avoid illegally releasing patient information [106]. Consistent training and evaluations are necessary for ensuring compliance. Acquiring explicit informed permission is crucial for safeguarding privacy. It is essential to provide patients with information on the use of their data and provide them with the autonomy to decline or retract their consent.

PM is an emerging strategy for treating and preventing diseases that provides tailored care by considering specific aspects such as an individual's genetic composition, environment, and lifestyle. The development has been hastened by technological breakthroughs such as ample data storage, sensor technology, and the IoT. Nevertheless, there are notable technical obstacles, namely, about the security and confidentiality of precision health data, such as the human genome. These issues are poorly understood and potentially jeopardize patients' electronic health records [107].

In the fields of life science and precision healthcare, regulatory innovation is essential. In 2020, the FDA approved 66% of new medications through expedited review processes. The Evidence Platform from Aetion backs drug approvals. By 2028, the global market for human microbiomes is anticipated to generate $1,598 million, providing new opportunities for illness prevention and treatment [108]. By 2025, the worldwide healthcare blockchain industry is anticipated to reach $5.6 billion, facilitating safer patient data exchange and better care coordination [109].

Ensuring patients' privacy is of utmost importance during AI assessment. It is essential to tell them about the storage and use of their data, get their permission *via* signed documents, and allow them to withdraw their consent at any given moment. The General Data Protection Regulation (GDPR) [110, 111] governs data privacy in Europe, guaranteeing openness, integrity, and the ability to alter one's decisions. AI assessment should be securely housed and maintained, with stringent access restrictions and the deletion of personal data, including both directly and indirectly associated data [112].

DISCUSSION

To enhance population health and lessen health inequalities, precision public health, akin to precision medicine, seeks to provide the correct intervention to the right population at the right time. Backed by the Gates Foundation, this project utilizes individual-level data and advanced scientific methods for precision treatment. This strategy combines vaccination acceptance, societal environment, personal medical history, genetic information, biological indicators, and variables contributing to the likelihood of experiencing adverse outcomes [113]. Mobile and social network technology can provide customized interventions. The efficacy of precision public health relies on addressing mathematical obstacles, accurately identifying the target group for the intervention, using appropriate data, and preventing unauthorized use of data.

Big medical data management presents issues for the healthcare sector since it might take years to analyze, link, and provide reliable diagnoses. AI is assisting enterprises in analyzing health information, streamlining examinations, and managing patient records. When implemented, AI solutions may enhance data processing and provide rapid insight into patterns, a task that can be difficult for people.

Precision healthcare, which integrates biomedical engineering and Artificial Intelligence, transforms medical interventions by improving diagnoses, tailoring treatments, and prioritizing patient-centered care. Nevertheless, the obstacles include ethical issues, legislative frameworks, and fair access to cutting-edge technology. The varied characteristics of healthcare data provide difficulties in assuring accurate representation and preventing biases in AI algorithms. Successfully incorporating precision healthcare into clinical operations requires a careful equilibrium between inventive ideas and feasible execution.

The adoption of healthcare relies heavily on the implementation of ethical AI since algorithms need to demonstrate high performance across a wide range of patient groups. Nevertheless, there is a potential danger of human biases being ingrained in algorithms, which are often constructed as opaque "black boxes" without transparency [114].

Life sciences start-ups are increasingly interested in PM because of its potential advantages, such as optimized resource use, enhanced therapeutic effectiveness, decreased occurrence of adverse medication responses, and better treatment compliance. By 2026, the worldwide market for PM is expected to be valued at USD 1.7 trillion [115].

The healthcare equity problem is of great importance since there are observed discrepancies in treatment and results based on different patient characteristics. Environmental issues, poverty, racism, and other issues have a detrimental effect on minority communities in the United States [116]. Genetics is a possible approach to mitigate health inequities. Still, it is essential not to overlook non-genetic elements significantly impacting people's health [117]. PM instruments may facilitate the advancement of precision public health.

Additionally, knowledge of quality improvement and patient-centeredness can contribute to equality efforts and increase communication and cultural competence among healthcare workers. Integrating information about genetic risk into clinical and public health tools may significantly enhance the ability to address health and healthcare disparities. It can also provide valuable insights for guiding practice and policy decisions to mitigate possible dangers associated with population-based genomic investigations [118]. The level of fairness may increase further if a growing number of patients choose precision medicine-based therapies under the right-to-try legislation [119]. Concentrating on the most frequently occurring disorders may exacerbate the disparity between individuals with prevalent diseases and other patient cohorts [120, 121]. An essential factor in resolving equity-related concerns is adopting a collaborative strategy involving clinicians and patients, with the active participation of technology specialists.

CONCLUSIONS

Precision health is an expanding discipline that uses AI to analyze health data, diagnose diseases at an early stage, and provide individualized preventive actions. Nevertheless, ethical considerations have prompted the development of national and international frameworks to ensure the responsible use of AI. The healthcare community is worried about misunderstandings regarding customized and precision medicine. Personalized medicine is a therapeutic approach that tailors treatment to a patient's specific features. Precision medicine, on the other hand, utilizes many sources of big data to create medications, vaccinations, and nutrition plans based on the illness's biological components. This technique improves treatment efficiency by incorporating genetic and molecular information into standard medical practice. Personalized medicine seeks to enhance healthcare by facilitating timely diagnoses for patients, while PM provides disease-focused services with a high level of detail utilizing various data sources.

FUTURE DIRECTIONS

In the future, one of the obstacles that precision healthcare systems must overcome is the variety of data and disparities in computer power and speed. To tackle these challenges, adversarial training, distributed training, trusted workers, federated learning frameworks, improved auditing systems, and other similar strategies may be utilized. Integrated efforts, leadership coordination, investment in digital infrastructure, and ongoing clinical staff upskilling are necessary for a successful deployment.

REFERENCES

[1] Collins FS, Varmus H. A new initiative on precision medicine. N Engl J Med 2015; 372(9): 793-5. [http://dx.doi.org/10.1056/NEJMp1500523] [PMID: 25635347]

[2] Duffy DJ. Problems, challenges and promises: perspectives on precision medicine. Brief Bioinform 2016; 17(3): 494-504. [http://dx.doi.org/10.1093/bib/bbv060] [PMID: 26249224]

[3] Schüssler-Fiorenza Rose SM, Contrepois K, Moneghetti KJ, *et al.* A longitudinal big data approach for precision health. Nat Med 2019; 25(5): 792-804. [http://dx.doi.org/10.1038/s41591-019-0414-6] [PMID: 31068711]

[4] Fu MR, Kurnat-Thoma E, Starkweather A, *et al.* Precision health: A nursing perspective. Int J Nurs Sci 2020; 7(1): 5-12. [http://dx.doi.org/10.1016/j.ijnss.2019.12.008] [PMID: 32099853]

[5] Precision health: improving health for each of us and all of us. CDC. 2020. Available from: https://www.cdc.gov/genomics/about/ precision_med.htm

[6] Hammond, Ray. 2020. The World In 2040—Future Health, Care & Well-Being. Available from: https://www.allianz-partners.com/en_US/press-and-media/reports/future-health-care-wellbeing.html

[7] Parimbelli E, Marini S, Sacchi L, Bellazzi R. Patient similarity for precision medicine: A systematic review. J Biomed Inform 2018; 83: 87-96.

[http://dx.doi.org/10.1016/j.jbi.2018.06.001] [PMID: 29864490]

[8] Kalouguina V, Wagner J. Challenges and Solutions for Integrating and Financing Personalized Medicine in Healthcare Systems: A Systematic Literature Review. J Risk Financ Manag 2020; 13(11): 283.
[http://dx.doi.org/10.3390/jrfm13110283]

[9] Gavan SP, Thompson AJ, Payne K. The economic case for precision medicine. Expert Rev Precis Med Drug Dev 2018; 3(1): 1-9.
[http://dx.doi.org/10.1080/23808993.2018.1421858] [PMID: 29682615]

[10] Available from: https://www.weforum.org/communities/precision-medicine/

[11] Available from: https://www.healthcareradius.in/clinical/treatment/precision-medicine-addressing-indias-health-challenge

[12] Ali A. Precision healthcare: integrating biomedical engineering and AI for tailored patient solutions. EasyChair Preprint. 2024 Feb 18;12171:13 p. Available from: https://easychair.org/publications/preprint/HHKn

[13] Available from: https://www.genome.gov/genetics-glossary/Precision-Healthcare

[14] Available from: https://www.usfhealthonline.com/resources/health-informatics/the-role-of-health-informatics-in-precision-medicine/

[15] Available from: https://medlineplus.gov/genetics/understanding/precisionmedicine/definition/

[16] Available from: https://health.ucdavis.edu/precision-medicine/what-is-precision-medicine.html

[17] Research BCC. Genomics: Technologies. Competitors, and Opportunities 2021.

[18] Jumper J, Evans R, Pritzel A, *et al.* Highly accurate protein structure prediction with AlphaFold. Nature 2021; 596(7873): 583-9.
[http://dx.doi.org/10.1038/s41586-021-03819-2] [PMID: 34265844]

[19] Polaris Market Research. Digital Health Market Share, Size, Trends, Industry Analysis Report. 2021.

[20] Sherman RE, Anderson SA, Dal Pan GJ, et al. Real-world evidence: what is it and what can it tell us? N Engl J Med. 2016 Dec 8; 375(23): 2293–7.
[http://dx.doi.org/10.1056/NEJMsb1609216] [PMID: 27959688]

[21] Foundation Medicine. Foundation One CDx. 2021.

[22] Quick J, Loman NJ, Duraffour S, *et al.* Real-time, portable genome sequencing for Ebola surveillance. Nature 2016; 530(7589): 228-32.
[http://dx.doi.org/10.1038/nature16996] [PMID: 26840485]

[23] Colijn C, Jones N, Johnston IG, Yaliraki S, Barahona M. Toward Precision Healthcare: Context and Mathematical Challenges. Front Physiol 2017; 8: 136.
[http://dx.doi.org/10.3389/fphys.2017.00136] [PMID: 28377724]

[24] Seymour CW, Gomez H, Chang CCH, *et al.* Precision medicine for all? Challenges and opportunities for a precision medicine approach to critical illness. Crit Care 2017; 21(1): 257.
[http://dx.doi.org/10.1186/s13054-017-1836-5] [PMID: 29047353]

[25] Bertsimas D, Kallus N, Weinstein AM, Zhuo YD. Personalized Diabetes Management Using Electronic Medical Records. Diabetes Care 2017; 40(2): 210-7.
[http://dx.doi.org/10.2337/dc16-0826] [PMID: 27920019]

[26] Bertsimas D, Orfanoudaki A, Weiner RB. Personalized treatment for coronary artery disease patients: a machine learning approach. Health Care Manage Sci 2020; 23(4): 482-506.
[http://dx.doi.org/10.1007/s10729-020-09522-4]

[27] Shea S, Hripcsak G. Accelerating the use of electronic health records in physician practices. N Engl J Med 2010; 362(3): 192-5.

[http://dx.doi.org/10.1056/NEJMp0910140] [PMID: 20089969]

[28] The Learning Healthcare System: Workshop Summary (Eds: Olsen L. A., Aisner D., McGinnis J. M.), The National Academies Collection: Reports funded by National Institutes of Health, Washington, DC: 2007.

[29] Friedman C. A broad-coverage natural language processing system. Proc AMIA Symp 2000; 270-4. [PMID: 11079887]

[30] Aronson AR. Effective mapping of biomedical text to the UMLS Metathesaurus: the MetaMap program. Proc AMIA Symp 2001; 17-21. [PMID: 11825149]

[31] Oniki TA, Zhuo N, Beebe CE, *et al.* Clinical element models in the SHARPn consortium. J Am Med Inform Assoc 2016; 23(2): 248-56. [http://dx.doi.org/10.1093/jamia/ocv134] [PMID: 26568604]

[32] Available from: https://www.cas.org/resources/cas-insights/dealing-challenges-drug-discovery#:~:text=Challenges%20such%20as%20rising%20costs,Are%20the%20current%20efforts%20successful%3F

[33] Available from: https://wintongibbons.com/infographic-precision-medicine-challenges-and-opportunities/

[34] Available from: https://www.lifebit.ai/blog/current-challenges-of-drug-discovery

[35] Available from: https://www.minfytech.com/ai-solutions-in-healthcare/

[36] Sanderson SC, Linderman MD, Suckiel SA, *et al.* Motivations, concerns and preferences of personal genome sequencing research participants: Baseline findings from the HealthSeq project. Eur J Hum Genet 2016; 24(1): 14-20. [http://dx.doi.org/10.1038/ejhg.2015.118] [PMID: 26036856]

[37] Ghafur S, Van Dael J, Leis M, Darzi A, Sheikh A. Public perceptions on data sharing: key insights from the UK and the USA. Lancet Digit Health 2020; 2(9): e444-6. [http://dx.doi.org/10.1016/S2589-7500(20)30161-8] [PMID: 32838250]

[38] Montgomery J. Data sharing and the idea of ownership. New Bioeth 2017; 23(1): 81-6. [http://dx.doi.org/10.1080/20502877.2017.1314893] [PMID: 28517982]

[39] Bernier A, Molnár-Gábor F, Knoppers BM, *et al.* Reconciling the biomedical data commons and the GDPR: three lessons from the EUCAN ELSI collaboratory. Eur J Hum Genet 2024; 32(1): 69-76. [http://dx.doi.org/10.1038/s41431-023-01403-y] [PMID: 37322132]

[40] Kong HJ. Managing unstructured big data in the healthcare system. Healthc Inform Res 2019; 25(1): 1-2. [http://dx.doi.org/10.4258/hir.2019.25.1.1] [PMID: 30788175]

[41] Savova GK, Danciu I, Alamudun F, *et al.* Use of Natural Language Processing to extract clinical cancer phenotypes from electronic medical records. Cancer Res 2019; 79(21): 5463-70. [http://dx.doi.org/10.1158/0008-5472.CAN-19-0579] [PMID: 31395609]

[42] Sweeney SM, Hamadeh HK, Abrams N, *et al.* Challenges to using big data in cancer. Cancer Res 2023; 83(8): 1175-82. [http://dx.doi.org/10.1158/0008-5472.CAN-22-1274] [PMID: 36625843]

[43] The Clinical Cancer Genome Task Team of the Global Alliance for Genomics and Health. Sharing clinical and genomic data on cancer — the need for global solutions. N Engl J Med. 2017 Jun 1;376: 2006–9. [http://dx.doi.org/10.1056/NEJMp1612254] [PMID: 28538124]

[44] Schuetz P, Aujesky D, Müller C, Müller B. Biomarker-guided personalised emergency medicine for all – hope for another hype? Swiss Med Wkly 2015; 145(708): w14079. [http://dx.doi.org/10.4414/smw.2015.14079] [PMID: 25695147]

[45] Available from: https://www.pwc.com/gx/en/issues/transformation/insights/transforming-precisio--health.html

[46] Available from: https://health.ucdavis.edu/precision-medicine/what-is-precision-medicine.html

[47] Available from: https://www.tevixmd.com/news-and-insights/understanding-patient-demographics-the-ultimate-guide-for-healthcare-providers

[48] Available from: https://medicine.iu.edu/expertise/precision-health/scientific-pillars

[49] Available from: https://archive.cdc.gov/www_cdc_gov/niosh/topics/exposome/default.html#:~:text=The%20exposome%20can%20be%20defined,%2C%20diet%2C%20lifestyle%2C%20etc

[50] Ryan K, Dockray S, Linehan C. A systematic review of tailored eHealth interventions for weight loss. Digit Health 2019; 5: 2055207619826685.
[http://dx.doi.org/10.1177/2055207619826685] [PMID: 30783535]

[51] Kostkova P. Grand challenges in digital health. Front Public Health 2015; 3: 134.
[http://dx.doi.org/10.3389/fpubh.2015.00134] [PMID: 26000272]

[52] Gambhir SS, Ge TJ, Vermesh O, Spitler R. Toward achieving precision health. Sci Transl Med 2018; 10(430): eaao3612.
[http://dx.doi.org/10.1126/scitranslmed.aao3612] [PMID: 29491186]

[53] Available from: https://www.precisionmedicine.columbia.edu/content/precision-medicine-patient-care

[54] Wang X. Gene mutation-based and specific therapies in precision medicine. J Cell Mol Med 2016; 20(4): 577-80.
[http://dx.doi.org/10.1111/jcmm.12722] [PMID: 26994883]

[55] Available from: https://vial.com/blog/articles/what-role-does-genetics-play-in-person-lized-medicine/?https://vial.com/blog/articles/what-role-does-genetics-p-ay-in-personalized-medicine/?utm_source=organic

[56] Zambelli-Weiner A. The Three Roles Precision Medicine Plays in Advancing Health Equity. Healthcare Information and Management Systems Society, Inc. 2021. Available from: https://www.himss.org/resources/three-roles-precision-medicine

[57] Mills MC, Rahal C. A scientometric review of genome-wide association studies. Commun Biol 2019; 2(1): 9.
[http://dx.doi.org/10.1038/s42003-018-0261-x] [PMID: 30623105]

[58] Callier S. The use of racial categories in precision medicine research. Ethn Dis 2019; 29 (Suppl.): 651-8.
[http://dx.doi.org/10.18865/ed.29.S3.651] [PMID: 31889770]

[59] Centers for Disease Control and Prevention. The U.S. Public Health Service Syphilis Study at Tuskegee 2022. Available from: https://www.cdc.gov/tuskegee/index.html

[60] Available from: https://www.healthviewx.com/advantages-disadvantages-precision-medicine/

[61] Available from: https://sengenics.com/blog/advancing-precision-medicine-emerging-trends-technologies/

[62] Available from: https://medicine.utah.edu/dbmi/aime/ai-and-precision

[63] Finlayson S.G., Bowers J.D., Ito J., Zittrain J.L., Beam L., Kohane I.S. Emerging vulnerabilities demand new conversations. Science (80) 2019; 363(6433): 1287–1290.

[64] Meskó B, Hetényi G, Győrffy Z. Will artificial intelligence solve the human resource crisis in healthcare? BMC Health Serv Res 2018; 18(1): 545.
[http://dx.doi.org/10.1186/s12913-018-3359-4] [PMID: 30001717]

[65] Arbelaez Ossa L, Starke G, Lorenzini G, Vogt JE, Shaw DM, Elger BS. Re-focusing explainability in medicine. Digit Health 2022; 8

[http://dx.doi.org/10.1177/20552076221074488] [PMID: 35173981]

[66] Dave D, Naik H, Singhal S, et al. Explainable AI meets healthcare: a study on heart disease dataset. arXiv [cs.LG]. 2020 Nov 6; arXiv:2011.03195. [http://dx.doi.org/10.48550/arXiv.2011.03195]

[67] 0. Arras L, Arjona-Medina J, Widrich M, et al. Explaining and interpreting LSTMs. In: Samek W, Montavon G, Vedaldi A, Hansen LK, Müller KR, eds. Explainable AI: Interpreting, Explaining and Visualizing Deep Learning. Springer International Publishing; 2019:211-238. [http://dx.doi.org/10.1007/978-3-030-28954-6_11]

[68] Oh S, Kim JH, Choi SW, Lee HJ, Hong J, Kwon SH. Physician confidence in artificial intelligence: an online mobile survey. J Med Internet Res 2019; 21(3): e12422. [http://dx.doi.org/10.2196/12422] [PMID: 30907742]

[69] Hernán MA. A definition of causal effect for epidemiological research. J Epidemiol Community Health 2004; 58(4): 265-71. [http://dx.doi.org/10.1136/jech.2002.006361] [PMID: 15026432]

[70] Edwards JK, Cole SR, Westreich D. All your data are always missing: Incorporating bias due to measurement error into the potential outcomes framework. Int J Epidemiol 2015; 44(4): 1452-9. [http://dx.doi.org/10.1093/ije/dyu272] [PMID: 25921223]

[71] Health IT Dashboard. Available from: https://dashboard.healthit.gov/quickstats/pages/physician-eh--adoption-trends.php

[72] Adler-Milstein J, Holmgren AJ, Kralovec P, Worzala C, Searcy T, Patel V. Electronic health record adoption in US hospitals: the emergence of a digital "advanced use" divide. J Am Med Inform Assoc 2017; 24(6): 1142-8. [http://dx.doi.org/10.1093/jamia/ocx080] [PMID: 29016973]

[73] Available from: https://www.techtarget.com/healthtechanalytics/news/366590097/Framework-t--Address-Algorithmic-Bias-in-Healthc-
re-A-
-
Models#:~:text=A%20growing%20body%20of%20research,negatively%2C%20impact%20health%20equity%20efforts

[74] Moja L, Polo Friz H, Capobussi M, *et al.* Effectiveness of a hospital-based computerized decision support system on clinician recommendations and patient outcomes: a randomized clinical trial. JAMA Netw Open 2019; 2(12): e1917094. [http://dx.doi.org/10.1001/jamanetworkopen.2019.17094] [PMID: 31825499]

[75] Tsopra R, Fernandez X, Luchinat C, *et al.* A framework for validating AI in precision medicine: considerations from the European ITFoC consortium. BMC Med Inform Decis Mak 2021; 21(1): 274. [http://dx.doi.org/10.1186/s12911-021-01634-3] [PMID: 34600518]

[76] Available from: https://www.pfizer.com/science/innovation/precision-medicine

[77] Bierman AS, Tinetti ME. Precision medicine to precision care: managing multimorbidity. Lancet 2016; 388(10061): 2721-3. [http://dx.doi.org/10.1016/S0140-6736(16)32232-2] [PMID: 27924764]

[78] Ward BW, Schiller JS. Prevalence of multiple chronic conditions among US adults: estimates from the National Health Interview Survey, 2010. Prev Chronic Dis 2013; 10: 120203. [http://dx.doi.org/10.5888/pcd10.120203] [PMID: 23618545]

[79] Rice TW, Wheeler AP, Thompson BT, *et al.* Initial trophic vs full enteral feeding in patients with acute lung injury: the EDEN randomized trial. JAMA 2012; 307(8): 795-803. [http://dx.doi.org/10.1001/jama.2012.137] [PMID: 22307571]

[80] Esteller M. Epigenetics in Cancer. N Engl J Med 2008; 358(11): 1148-59. [http://dx.doi.org/10.1056/NEJMra072067] [PMID: 18337604]

[81] Lichtenstein P, Holm NV, Verkasalo PK, *et al.* Environmental and heritable factors in the causation of cancer--analyses of cohorts of twins from Sweden, Denmark, and Finland. N Engl J Med 2000; 343(2): 78-85.
[http://dx.doi.org/10.1056/NEJM200007133430201] [PMID: 10891514]

[82] Available from: https://sanogenetics.com/resources/blog/what-are-the-economic-implications-of-precision-medicine#:~:text=Astonishingly%2C%20the%20precision%20approach%20was,with%20R%26D%20were%20significantly%20reduced

[83] Available from: https://www.himss.org/resources/predictive-medicine-advancing-healthcare-through-better-data-governance

[84] Insel TR. The NIMH research domain criteria (RDoC) project: precision medicine for psychiatry. Am J Psychiatry 2014; 171(4): 395-7.
[http://dx.doi.org/10.1176/appi.ajp.2014.14020138] [PMID: 24687194]

[85] Available from: https://handwiki.org/wiki/Philosophy:Generalization_(learning)

[86] Parker LS. Ethical considerations in precision medicine. In: Bydon M, editor. The new era of precision medicine. Academic Press; 2024. p. 143–72. doi: 10.1016/B978-0-443-13963-5.00002-9. Available from: https://www.sciencedirect.com/science/article/pii/B9780443139635000029

[87] Xu X, Hu J, Lyu X, Huang H, Cheng X. Exploring the Interdisciplinary Nature of Precision Medicine:Network Analysis and Visualization. JMIR Med Inform 2021; 9(1): e23562.
[http://dx.doi.org/10.2196/23562] [PMID: 33427681]

[88] Available from: https://www.paloaltonetworks.in/cyberpedia/ai-explainability

[89] Patty, Buttner, et al. "Healthcare Data Governance - Ahima." Healthcare Data Governance Practice Brief, AHIMA, Jan. 2022. Available from: https://www.ahima.org/media/pmcb0fr5/healthcare-dat--governance-practic

[90] Hekler E, Tiro JA, Hunter CM, Nebeker C. Precision health: the role of the social and behavioral sciences in advancing the vision. Ann Behav Med 2020; 54(11): 805-26.
[http://dx.doi.org/10.1093/abm/kaaa018] [PMID: 32338719]

[91] Solar O, Irwin A. A conceptual framework for action on the social determinants of health. World Health Organization. 2010. Available from: http://hdl.handle.net/1903/23135

[92] Available from: https://www.jax.org/personalized-medicine/precision-medicine-and-you/what-is-precision-medicine#

[93] Available from: https://en.wikipedia.org/wiki/Personalized_medicine

[94] Patrinos GP, Sarhangi N, Sarrami B, Khodayari N, Larijani B, Hasanzad M. Using ChatGPT to predict the future of personalized medicine. Pharmacogenomics J 2023; 23(6): 178-84.
[http://dx.doi.org/10.1038/s41397-023-00316-9] [PMID: 37726551]

[95] Available from: https://hoagconciergemedicine.com/personalized-medicine/

[96] Mehar Sahu, Rohan Gupta, Rashmi K. Ambasta, Pravir Kumar, Artificial Intelligence and Machine Learning in precision medicine: A paradigm shift in big data analysis, Progress in Molecular Biology and Translational Science, Academic Press, Volume 190, Issue 1, 2022, Pages 57-100, ISSN 1877-1173, ISBN 9780323997843.
[http://dx.doi.org/10.1016/bs.pmbts.2022.03.002]

[97] Baiardini I. Enrico Heffler, The Patient-Centered Decision System as per the 4Ps of Precision Medicine, Implementing Precision Medicine in Best Practices of Chronic Airway Diseases. Academic Press 2019; pp. 147-51.
[http://dx.doi.org/10.1016/B978-0-12-813471-9.00024-4]

[98] Tran TQB, du Toit C, Padmanabhan S. Artificial intelligence in healthcare—the road to precision medicine. J Hosp Manag Health Policy 2021; 5: 29.

[http://dx.doi.org/10.21037/jhmhp-20-132]

[99] Koleva-Kolarova R, Szilberhorn L, Zelei T, *et al.* Financial incentives to promote personalized medicine in Europe: An overview and guidance for implementation. Per Med 2023; 20(4): 305-19. [http://dx.doi.org/10.2217/pme-2022-0145] [PMID: 37623911]

[100] Regier DA, Pollard S, McPhail M, Bubela T, Hanna TP, Ho C, Lim HJ, Chan K, Peacock SJ and Weymann D, 2022. A perspective on life-cycle health technology assessment and real-world evidence for precision oncology in Canada. npj Precision Oncology 6(1), 76.

[101] Leopold JA, Loscalzo J. Emerging Role of Precision Medicine in Cardiovascular Disease. Circ Res 2018; 122(9): 1302-15. [http://dx.doi.org/10.1161/CIRCRESAHA.117.310782] [PMID: 29700074]

[102] Dewey FE, Pan S, Wheeler MT, Quake SR, Ashley EA. DNA Sequencing. Circulation 2012; 125(7): 931-44. [http://dx.doi.org/10.1161/CIRCULATIONAHA.110.972828] [PMID: 22354974]

[103] Dewey FE, Pan S, Wheeler MT, et al. DNA sequencing: clinical applications of new DNA sequencing technologies. Circulation. 2012 Feb 21; 125(7): 931–44. [http://dx.doi.org/10.1161/CIRCULATIONAHA.110.972828]

[104] Selleck MJ, Senthil M, Wall NR. Making Meaningful Clinical Use of Biomarkers. Biomark Insights 2017; 12 [http://dx.doi.org/10.1177/1177271917715236] [PMID: 28659713]

[105] Hasin Y, Seldin M, Lusis A. Multi-omics approaches to disease. Genome Biol 2017; 18(1): 83. [http://dx.doi.org/10.1186/s13059-017-1215-1] [PMID: 28476144]

[106] Bludau I, Aebersold R. Proteomic and interactomic insights into the molecular basis of cell functional diversity. Nat Rev Mol Cell Biol 2020; 21(6): 327-40. [http://dx.doi.org/10.1038/s41580-020-0231-2] [PMID: 32235894]

[107] Ramkumar Thirunavukkarasu, George Priya Doss C, Gnanasambandan R, Mohanraj Gopikrishnan, Venkatesh Palanisamy, Towards computational solutions for precision medicine based big data healthcare system using Deep Learning models: A review, Computers in Biology and Medicine, Volume 149,2022,106020, ISSN 0010-825, [http://dx.doi.org/10.1016/j.compbiomed.2022.106020]

[108] Manickam P, Mariappan SA, Murugesan SM, *et al.* Artificial intelligence (AI) and the Internet of Medical Things (IoMT) assisted biomedical systems for intelligent healthcare. Biosensors (Basel) 2022; 12(8): 562. [http://dx.doi.org/10.3390/bios12080562] [PMID: 35892459]

[109] Sollins H. Circulation 2003; 108: 915. [http://dx.doi.org/10.1161/01.CIR.0000085720.65685.90] [PMID: 12939241]

[110] Available from: https://onlineacademiccommunity.uvic.ca/isot/2022/11/28/security-and-privacy-for-precision-health/

[111] Georgiou A, Magrabi F, Hyppönen H, *et al.* The safe and effective use of shared data underpinned by stakeholder engagement and evaluation practice. Yearb Med Inform 2018; 27(1): 025-8. [http://dx.doi.org/10.1055/s-0038-1641194] [PMID: 29681039]

[112] U data protection rules. European Commission - European Commission. Available from: https://ec.europa.eu/commission/priorities/justice-and-fundamental-rights/d-ta-protection/2018-reform-eu-data-protection-rules/eu-data-protection-rules_en

[113] Doel T, Shakir DI, Pratt R, *et al.* GIFT-Cloud: A data sharing and collaboration platform for medical imaging research. Comput Methods Programs Biomed 2017; 139: 181-90. [http://dx.doi.org/10.1016/j.cmpb.2016.11.004] [PMID: 28187889]

[114] Grand View Research. Human Microbiome Market Size, Share & Trends Analysis Report. 2021.

[115] BIS Research. Global Healthcare Blockchain Technology Market. 2021.

[116] Available from: https://jnjinnovation.com/news/blog-post/precision-health-medicine--opportunities-challenges

[117] CDC Health Disparities and Inequalities Report – United States, 2013. MMWR 2013; 62 (Suppl. 3): 1-189.

[118] Sankar P, Cho MK, Condit CM, *et al.* Genetic research and health disparities. JAMA 2004; 291(24): 2985-9.
[http://dx.doi.org/10.1001/jama.291.24.2985] [PMID: 15213210]

[119] Cooper LA, Ortega AN, Ammerman AS, *et al.* Calling for a bold new vision of health disparities intervention research. Am J Public Health 2015; 105(S3) (Suppl. 3): S374-6.
[http://dx.doi.org/10.2105/AJPH.2014.302386] [PMID: 25905830]

[120] Jacob JA. Questions of safety and fairness are raised as the right-to-try movement gains steam. JAMA 2015; 314(8): 758-60.
[http://dx.doi.org/10.1001/jama.2015.7691] [PMID: 26244653]

[121] Available from: https://law.pace.edu/sites/default/files/PECC/Wind_ToolKit_Updates_Chap8_TOP_12JULY2011_TOP_19OCT2011.pdf

CHAPTER 2

Achieving Precision in Healthcare: A Path Forward

Darshna M. Joshi[1,*]

[1] *Department of Instrumentation and Control Engineering, Government Polytechnic, Ahmedabad, Gujarat, India*

Abstract: Precision healthcare is an approach aimed at delivering personalized medical treatments tailored to the unique needs of individuals. Personalized medicine, also known as precision medicine, is a healthcare approach that considers genetics, lifestyle, and environmental factors, classifying individuals based on their medical histories. Its goal is to prevent disease and develop target-based solutions for various medical conditions. Serving as a predictive model, this model aids in developing medical solutions customized explicitly to the ailment at concern. The practical implementation of this model requires collecting and analyzing large datasets. This presents a global challenge for the effective implementation of precision medicine. It also raises ethical, social, and legal concerns, including the importance of safeguarding patients' private health information. Millions of dollars in funding are required for precision medicine to be implemented successfully over the long term. Another significant issue that must be addressed when addressing the concept of precision medicine is the necessity for trained professionals. Large datasets can be handled due to contemporary technologies like machine learning and artificial intelligence. Additionally, researchers working together to improve the results are advantageous. Shortly, patients and healthcare professionals can look forward to the greatest tailored therapies and treatments with the advancements in modern medicine. This chapter addresses the challenges faced in effectively implementing precision medicine healthcare and discusses solutions for efficient healthcare delivery to improve patient outcomes for disease prevention.

Keywords: Advancements, Challenges, Disease prevention, Modern technology, Precision medicine, Personalized healthcare.

INTRODUCTION

Precision healthcare is an emerging approach that focuses on treating and preventing diseases. This approach considers the unique characteristics of each

* **Corresponding author Darshna M. Joshi:** Department of Instrumentation and Control Engineering, Government Polytechnic, Ahmedabad, Gujarat, India; E-mail: darshna.joshi91@gmail.com

Neeraj Gupta, Abdelhameed Ibrahim, Bhavesh Vyas & Shobhna Jeet (Eds.)

patient, tailoring treatment to enhance accuracy and effectiveness. The term "precision medicine" was coined by the "National Research Council report", which emphasized individual characteristics-based healthcare. All medicines are developed with precision in mind [1]. However, the precision healthcare approach is focused on personal traits like specific biological modifications, gene structure or regulation, transcription, and molecular signaling pathways. Fig. (**1**) illustrates the relationship between genetic and environmental factors that influence human health, which is essential for developing personalized healthcare solutions. Precision medicine allows doctors and researchers to classify each line of treatment for a particular class of people based on their response to the treatment. It is a "different for all" approach, where the cure for a disease is based on individual signs rather than a "one fits all" approach. A widely recognized example is blood donation, where compatibility between donor and recipient blood types is rigorously verified to prevent complications [2 - 5].

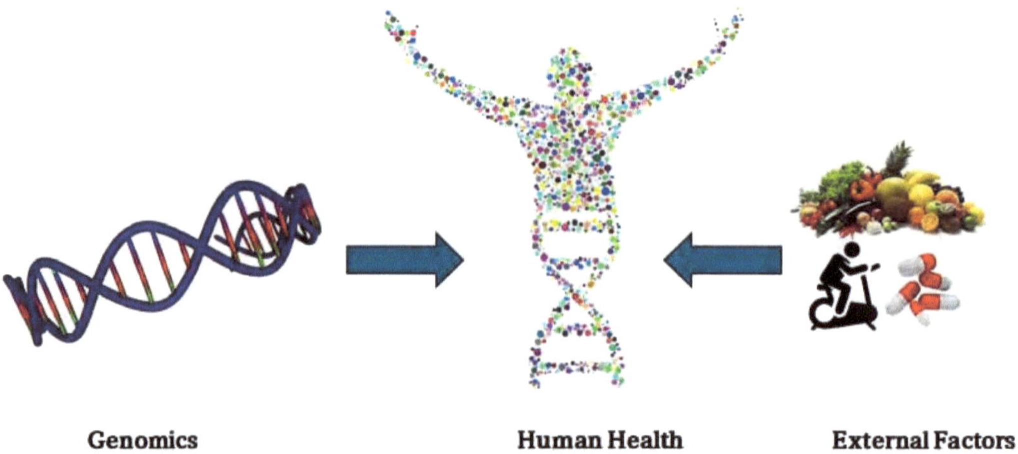

Fig. (1). Personalized healthcare: Relational factors.

The goal of precision medicine thus requires a large set of accurate data that can be analyzed to treat an individual precisely. Target-based medicinal treatment would benefit from this kind of data, which can help eradicate diseases like cancer and diabetes. Fig. (**2**) illustrates the flow of implementing complete personalized healthcare. Collecting large data sets with legal, ethical, and social guidelines is challenging. Advanced computational tools and techniques are required to ensure precise health information is collected. Artificial intelligence and machine learning can bridge data analysis for precise outcomes based on available data sets. For the same, funding agencies should come forward to boost the process of precision healthcare. All these insights aid in opting for a global collaboration that could result in health innovations for precision medicine healthcare. The full potential of digital data can only be utilized if we think globally without any regional or financial boundaries. The medical field is shifting from conventional treatments to target-based treatment based on patients' information, which can bring out more precise healthcare decisions [1 - 15].

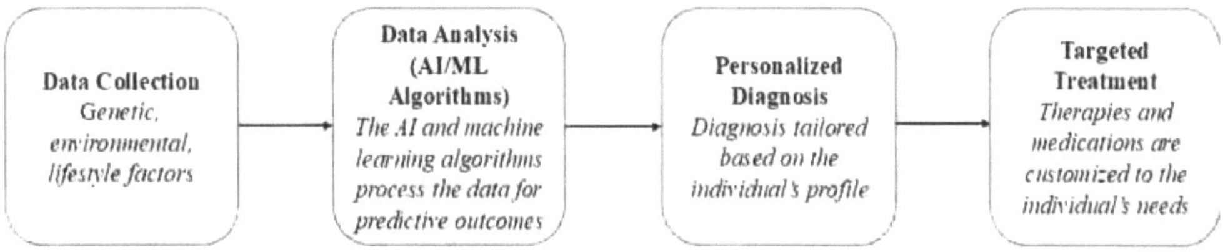

Fig. (2). Personalized healthcare flowchart.

We begin by discussing the objectives of implementing precision healthcare. We next address significant challenges to precision medicine in classifying individuals based on their history for a future personalized approach for specific treatments. We discussed the challenge of handling large datasets and using advanced computational tools to analyze the data precisely and promptly. Also, the funding challenges are elaborated on, and the availability and possibilities are discussed. Finally, we discuss a road map to achieve objectives while considering the challenges of transforming medical care from one for all to individual personalized healthcare.

OBJECTIVES

Advances in medical technology have improved the understanding of the link between DNA sequences and the underlying causes of diseases. The success rate of gene therapies is improving, but it is not cost-effective. Precision healthcare is the latest trending approach for dealing with patients' health *via* individually tailored therapies and thus extends the lifespan [2 - 6]. Based on the lifestyle and other factors like cultural, economic, and environmental, precision healthcare helps patients achieve optimal health. Integrating genomic, clinical, and outcome data would enhance the individual's health. The following are the objectives of precision healthcare [8, 16 - 19].

- Extensive data collection of individuals' health based on various factors.
- Identify the most suitable care for each patient.
- Determine the changes in the genetic factors that lead to the disease when the conditions are undiagnosed.
- Prescribe medications that can avoid serious side effects.
- Identify the lifestyle, cultural, and environmental factors that can lessen the side effects of medications and dosages.

- Provide a proactive response to the causes behind the diseases.
- Identify risk factors individually and provide a customized preventive screening.
- Schedule vaccination based on personalized health data.
- Activate strategies that could detect disease biomarkers early to provide timely medications.
- Implement personalized nutrition plans to improve individuals' lifestyles.
- Develop personalized dietary plans and nutritional guidelines based on genetic and metabolic profiles.
- Optimize post-operative care plans based on individual genetic susceptibility.
- Develop customized rehabilitation programs for speedy recovery.
- Develop customized protocols for organ transplantation to minimize the risk of rejection.
- Enhance precise personalized pain management plans based on the individual's database.
- Customize age-based plans for diseases that come with ageing.

RATIONALE FOR OBJECTIVE SELECTION

The objectives outlined in this chapter were selected to comprehensively represent the essential elements required to implement precision healthcare successfully. The foundation of this approach lies in extensive data collection, which is vital for tailoring healthcare to individual needs. Without comprehensive genetic, environmental, cultural, and lifestyle data, healthcare systems cannot accurately assess risks, diagnose conditions early, or develop targeted interventions. Thus, objectives related to personalized screenings, early biomarker detection, and proactive disease prevention reflect the need to shift from reactive to predictive healthcare models. Similarly, goals such as identifying the most suitable care for each patient and prescribing medications that minimize adverse side effects are crucial for ensuring treatment effectiveness and patient safety, which are core goals of precision medicine.

Incorporating personalized dietary and vaccination plans further enhances the preventative nature of care, especially for populations at higher risk due to age or pre-existing conditions. Objectives focused on optimizing post-operative care and rehabilitation, as well as organ transplantation compatibility, emphasize the importance of precision throughout the patient journey, not just in diagnosis or medication. Moreover, the customization of pain management plans and protocols for ageing individuals acknowledges that treatment response varies significantly with age, requiring adjustments in care strategies. These objectives also recognize that non-genetic factors, such as socioeconomic status and environmental conditions, play a substantial role in health outcomes and must be integrated into personalized healthcare planning.

Collectively, these objectives align with global trends in precision medicine and respond to the pressing challenges in healthcare delivery, namely, rising chronic disease burdens, ageing populations, and the need for cost-effective, outcome-oriented interventions. Each selected objective contributes to building a framework where technology, data science, and personalized medical insights converge to provide reactive care and informed, proactive, and preventative healthcare solutions. These objectives aim to improve long-term patient outcomes, enhance the quality of life, and optimize resource allocation across healthcare systems by focusing on individual variability and leveraging modern tools like AI and genomics.

CHALLENGES

Precision healthcare faces numerous challenges. One of the most essential things is collecting and handling large amounts of data while keeping ethical and security concerns in mind. Even if the data is collected, its analysis is another tedious task to be completed, as interoperability between the data and the healthcare database is important. The ethical and security challenges surrounding patient data use remain significant concerns that researchers must address. Inaccuracy in data and response time plays a vital role. However, the advancement of precision treatment faces a barrier if the data about the target therapy takes longer. Healthcare professionals and researchers must receive specialized training in collecting and analyzing large datasets, as these skills are critical for realizing the full potential of precision healthcare. Specifically, if Artificial intelligence and Machine learning algorithms are used for handling and analyzing the data, precision in healthcare could be achieved more effectively. For the same, healthcare professionals should be trained and equipped to use the plans generated by algorithms more efficiently [11, 19, 20].

Another challenge is to identify the relevant genetic factor responsible for a particular disease, for which the cost and time for genetic testing and implementation pose a hurdle. At the same time, integrating non-genetic factors like cultural and socioeconomic factors while making healthcare decisions is challenging. Also, the nature of the disease needs to be understood so that an effective modification can be carried out in the lifestyle and other factors [7, 8, 19 - 23].

Furthermore, it is critical to overcome the vaccine hesitancy from individuals, as a personalized vaccine could lead to an effective solution in various diseases, even if it is a pandemic. The risk and side effects associated with the same can be lessened. For the same reason, it is difficult to develop algorithms or biomarkers that can help detect diseases at a very early stage. This can be done by providing personalized nutrition recommendations based on genetic and environmental factors. Developing protocols to be followed while making any surgical decision, as well as even after the operations are carried out, after going through the profile of an individual's genetic and other factors, is essential. Establishing rehabilitation centers for training healthcare workers and the individual traits group is a major challenge. If we talk about another challenge, organ transplantation needs personalized healthcare on a very high level; compatibility with the donor's organ is important for success. The same is true for the pain sensitivity of individuals to various medications based on profile and biomarkers [1, 7, 8, 19, 20, 22].

Of all these challenges, ageing is the most challenging. In such cases, the healthcare workforce needs to be specifically trained to provide personalized medications to adults based on lifestyle, genetic, and environmental factors.

The intricacy of precision healthcare necessitates solutions such as technical developments and collaborative interdisciplinary research to accomplish the goals effectively.

SOLUTIONS

The challenges discussed above can be addressed with a multifaceted approach based on advanced technology, ethical guidelines, and training programs for healthcare professionals. It is very important to note that just like personalized healthcare treats patients based on individual traits, solutions may be effective based on various personalized factors.

The challenge of collecting and handling data can be addressed by the implementation of robust policies on data management, keeping in mind the ethical guidelines as well as the security concerns of the patients. The development of standardized formats for data would provide a seamless integration of data across various healthcare systems globally. As mentioned, these large datasets can be handled by analyzing software running machine learning and artificial intelligence algorithms [24 - 30]. Based on standard patterns of the data, predictions about health can be made in advance. A collaboration between data handling agencies and healthcare professionals would enhance the interpretation of the outcome from the data. Data protection regulations in the world need to be made much stronger if such sensitive data is to be analyzed. Prompt decision-making in precision healthcare is very important; for the same reason, computing facilities need to be advanced for interoperability of the critical health information [5, 7, 13 - 15, 19].

The challenge associated with genetic testing can be addressed by developing cost-effective institutions that can train genetic researchers, healthcare professionals, and various drug-making companies to develop target-based therapies. Similarly, the challenges associated with providing personalized healthcare to ageing individuals could be solved by the development of telemedicine and digital healthcare *via* remote data monitoring. Surgical and transplantation decisions could be personalized if surgeons, geneticists, and rehabilitation specialists come together while making decisions. Organ matching algorithms could be developed on the basis of genetic compatibility using various computational tools and techniques to handle real-time data [24, 25, 28 - 31]. Along with genetic factors, non-genetic factors like lifestyle, environmental, and socioeconomic factors could also be addressed by updating the existing health records. Vaccine hesitancy is a significant challenge that could be addressed by launching various target-based campaigns for individuals in public health. For the same, a customized nutrition plan could be provided digitally to reach the world by collaborating with dietitians, genetic researchers, and nutritionists [32 - 41].

Effective implementation of all these solutions requires successful collaboration between healthcare professionals, researchers, ethical and security policy makers, technologists, and patients' advocacy groups. If the challenges are addressed systematically, precision healthcare can provide personalized treatment based on individual patient needs.

POLICY RECOMMENDATIONS FOR PRECISION HEALTHCARE

Several policies must be implemented to successfully implement precision healthcare and ensure that it reaches its full potential. These recommendations focus on overcoming barriers such as data management, ethical concerns, and resource allocation while also encouraging global collaboration to foster innovation and enhance patient outcomes [42 - 44].

Create Global Standards for Data Management and Protection

One of the most pressing needs for precision healthcare is the creation of universal standards for how patient data is collected, stored, and shared. Data from genetic tests, medical records, and other sources is essential for the success of personalized treatments, but it must be managed carefully to ensure privacy and security. Policymakers should work to establish international standards that not only guarantee data interoperability across different healthcare systems but also ensure patient confidentiality.

Global cooperation between healthcare institutions, technology providers, and governments will be crucial to achieve this. Laws protecting sensitive health information should be strengthened, and patients must be given clear and transparent options about how their data is used. This will protect privacy and build trust, encouraging more people to participate in data-sharing initiatives that are vital for the future of precision healthcare.

Increase Funding for Research and Technological Development

For precision healthcare to move forward, substantial funding must be directed toward research into genomic medicine, data science, and AI-driven healthcare technologies. Governments must allocate more resources for research into affordable genetic testing, AI-based diagnostics, and other technologies supporting personalized treatments. This should be a collaborative effort, with governments working alongside private companies and research institutions to pool resources and tackle the challenges together.

Support for public-private partnerships can also drive innovation, making cutting-edge treatments and technologies more accessible to patients. The goal is to reduce the high costs of precision medicine and make it available to a broader population. Public investment in genomics, bioinformatics, and related fields is essential for pushing the boundaries of medical research and delivering personalized therapies tailored to individual patients.

Develop Comprehensive Training Programs for Healthcare Professionals

The implementation of precision medicine requires healthcare professionals to be well-versed in the latest advances in genomics, data analysis, and AI. Policymakers should prioritize developing specialized training programs for healthcare providers focusing on understanding and applying personalized medicine approaches. This includes training on how to analyze and interpret large datasets, use machine learning algorithms in clinical settings, and incorporate genetic data into patient care.

Moreover, bioinformatics training is critical for clinicians who must interpret complex genetic information to provide personalized treatment recommendations. By integrating these skills into medical curricula and offering ongoing professional development, healthcare systems can ensure that professionals are prepared for the demands of precision medicine.

Strengthen Ethical Guidelines to Ensure Fair and Responsible Use of Data

As genetic and health data use becomes more widespread in precision medicine, ethical concerns are becoming more pronounced. Policymakers must establish clear guidelines for the ethical use of personal health information. This includes ensuring that patients are fully informed about the collection and use of their data and that consent processes are transparent and respected.

Ethical guidelines must address equity issues in addition to data privacy. Policies must ensure that personalized healthcare advances are available to the affluent and accessible to all populations, including underserved communities. Ensuring that precision medicine is implemented fairly will help prevent disparities in healthcare access and outcomes.

Foster Global Collaboration Through Research Networks

Precision healthcare is an interdisciplinary field that requires collaboration between geneticists, clinicians, bioinformaticians, AI specialists, and other professionals. To foster innovation, policymakers should encourage the formation of global research consortia that allow researchers from different countries to share data and insights. This will lead to a more comprehensive understanding of how genetic, environmental, and lifestyle factors influence health and how precision medicine can address these factors.

These collaborative networks will also help address health disparities by ensuring that research reflects diverse populations. Policies should promote the creation of global data-sharing platforms to facilitate collaborative efforts across borders, enabling scientists and clinicians to work together on solving complex healthcare challenges.

Increase Public Engagement and Awareness of Precision Healthcare

Public engagement is crucial for precision healthcare to gain widespread adoption. People need to understand the benefits of personalized medicine and how it can improve their health. Policymakers should support public awareness campaigns that explain precision medicine in clear, accessible language. These campaigns can help demystify the concept and show the practical ways it can be used to prevent disease, reduce side effects, and deliver better health outcomes.

Moreover, as personalized medicine evolves, resistance or hesitancy may exist, particularly around genetic testing and AI-driven decisions. Public health campaigns should address these concerns, providing evidence that personalized medicine is safe and highly effective in treating diseases like cancer, diabetes, and heart disease.

Overhaul Legal and Regulatory Frameworks

The legal landscape surrounding precision medicine must adapt to the new realities of personalized healthcare. Intellectual property laws, regulatory processes, and liability issues must all be revisited to support integrating new technologies. For instance, laws regarding the ownership of genetic data and the use of AI algorithms in medical decisions should be clarified.

Regulatory agencies should work more closely with healthcare providers and technology companies to streamline approval processes for genetic therapies and AI-based diagnostic tools. This would ensure that patients have quick access to innovative treatments without compromising safety.

Invest in Healthcare Infrastructure and Technology Access

Access to precision healthcare will be limited unless healthcare systems are equipped with the necessary infrastructure. Governments should invest in upgrading medical facilities with the latest diagnostic technologies and ensure that healthcare providers have the tools to handle large datasets effectively. This may involve integrating AI-powered diagnostic tools, genetic sequencing platforms, and electronic health records that are optimized for precision medicine.

Telemedicine and digital health platforms also play a critical role in expanding access to personalized care, especially in rural or underserved areas. Investment in these technologies will ensure that even patients who live in remote locations can benefit from precision healthcare.

CONCLUDING REMARKS

Precision healthcare decision-making dominates the world over conventional healthcare systems if followed correctly. Although various challenges are associated with effectively implementing precision healthcare for personalized medicine, solutions always come. The most crucial point is the collaboration of healthcare individuals—researchers, geneticists, patients, data analysts, surgeons, policymakers, and whatnot. So, at present, every stakeholder needs to be armed with precision healthcare knowledge so that successful AI and ML applications can be made on large datasets for enhanced target-based health predictions, which need strong data handling platforms. The stakeholders' training is much needed for the successful implementation of precision healthcare.

REFERENCES

[1] Toward precision medicine: Building a knowledge network for biomedical research and a new taxonomy of disease. 2012. Epub ahead of print 2012. [http://dx.doi.org/10.17226/13284]

[2] Collins F. A new initiative on precision medicine. N Engl J Med; 363. [http://dx.doi.org/10.1056/NEJMp1500523]

[3] Ashley EA. The precision medicine initiative: a new national effort. JAMA 2015; 313(21): 2119-20. [http://dx.doi.org/10.1001/jama.2015.3595] [PMID: 25928209]

[4] Ghitza UE. A commentary on 'A new initiative on precision medicine'. Front Psychiatry 2015; 6: 88. [http://dx.doi.org/10.3389/fpsyt.2015.00088] [PMID: 26106336]

[5] Collins FS, Varmus H. A new initiative on precision medicine. N Engl J Med 2015; 372(9): 793-5. [http://dx.doi.org/10.1056/NEJMp1500523] [PMID: 25635347]

[6] Desmond-Hellmann S. Toward precision medicine: a new social contract? Sci Transl Med 2012; 4(129): 129ed3. [http://dx.doi.org/10.1126/scitranslmed.3003473] [PMID: 22496543]

[7] Adams SA, Petersen C. Precision medicine: opportunities, possibilities, and challenges for patients and providers. J Am Med Inform Assoc 2016; 23(4): 787-90. [http://dx.doi.org/10.1093/jamia/ocv215] [PMID: 26977101]

[8] Seymour CW, Gomez H, Chang CCH, *et al.* Precision medicine for all? Challenges and opportunities for a precision medicine approach to critical illness. Crit Care 2017; 21(1): 257. [http://dx.doi.org/10.1186/s13054-017-1836-5] [PMID: 29047353]

[9] Roberts MC, Fohner AE, Landry L, *et al.* Advancing precision public health using human genomics: examples from the field and future research opportunities. Genome Med 2021; 13(1): 97. [http://dx.doi.org/10.1186/s13073-021-00911-0] [PMID: 34074326]

[10] Nussinov R, Jang H, Nir G, Tsai CJ, Cheng F. A new precision medicine initiative at the dawn of exascale computing. Signal Transduct Target Ther 2021; 6(1): 3. [http://dx.doi.org/10.1038/s41392-020-00420-3] [PMID: 33402669]

[11] Chen GT, Geschwind DH. Challenges and opportunities for precision medicine in neurodevelopmental disorders. Adv Drug Deliv Rev 2022; 191: 114564. [http://dx.doi.org/10.1016/j.addr.2022.114564] [PMID: 36183905]

[12] Olson MV. Precision medicine at the crossroads. Hum Genomics 2017; 11(1): 23. [http://dx.doi.org/10.1186/s40246-017-0119-1] [PMID: 29020978]

[13] U.S. Food and Drug Administration. FDA's Role in a New Era of Medical Product Development. Paving W Pers Med.

[14] Kaul KL. Preparing pathology for precision medicine: challenges and opportunities. Virchows Arch 2017; 471(2): 141-6. [http://dx.doi.org/10.1007/s00428-017-2141-z] [PMID: 28512674]

[15] Lamberti MJ, Wilkinson M, Peña Y, et al. Preparing for precision medicine. Contract Pharma. Epub ahead of print 2018. [http://dx.doi.org/10.1056/NEJMp1114866]

[16] Joyner MJ, Paneth N. Promises, promises, and precision medicine. J Clin Invest 2019; 129(3): 946-8. [http://dx.doi.org/10.1172/JCI126119] [PMID: 30688663]

[17] Fu MR, Kurnat-Thoma E, Starkweather A, *et al.* Precision health: A nursing perspective. Int J Nurs Sci 2020; 7(1): 5-12. [http://dx.doi.org/10.1016/j.ijnss.2019.12.008] [PMID: 32099853]

[18] Panesar A. What Is Precision Health? In: Precision Health and Artificial Intelligence. 2023, pp. 19–45. [http://dx.doi.org/10.1007/978-1-4842-9162-7_2]

[19] Panesar A. Risks and Ethical Challenges of Precision Health. In: Precision Health and Artificial Intelligence. 2023. Epub ahead of print 2023. [http://dx.doi.org/10.1007/978-1-4842-9162-7_5]

[20] Naithani N, Atal AT, Tilak TVSVGK, Vasudevan B, Misra P, Sinha S. Precision medicine: Uses and challenges. Med J Armed Forces India 2021; 77(3): 258-65. [http://dx.doi.org/10.1016/j.mjafi.2021.06.020] [PMID: 34305277]

[21] Wang ZG, Zhang L, Zhao WJ. Definition and application of precision medicine. Chinese Journal of

Traumatology - English Edition; 19. Epub ahead of print 2016. [http://dx.doi.org/10.1016/j.cjtee.2016.04.005]

[22] Pelter MN, Druz RS. Precision medicine: Hype or hope? Trends Cardiovasc Med 2024; 34(2): 120-5. [http://dx.doi.org/10.1016/j.tcm.2022.11.001] [PMID: 36375778]

[23] De Maria Marchiano R, Di Sante G, Piro G, *et al.* Translational research in the era of precision medicine: Where we are and where we will go. J Pers Med 2021; 11(3): 216. [http://dx.doi.org/10.3390/jpm11030216] [PMID: 33803592]

[24] Quazi S. RETRACTED ARTICLE: Artificial intelligence and machine learning in precision and genomic medicine. Med Oncol 2022; 39(8): 120. [http://dx.doi.org/10.1007/s12032-022-01711-1] [PMID: 35704152]

[25] Martínez-García M, Hernández-Lemus E. Data Integration Challenges for Machine Learning in Precision Medicine. Front Med (Lausanne) 2022; 8: 784455. [http://dx.doi.org/10.3389/fmed.2021.784455] [PMID: 35145977]

[26] Lee S, Lam SH, Hernandes Rocha TA, *et al.* Machine Learning and Precision Medicine in Emergency Medicine: The Basics. Cureus 2021; 13(9): e17636. [http://dx.doi.org/10.7759/cureus.17636] [PMID: 34646684]

[27] MacEachern SJ, Forkert ND. Machine learning for precision medicine. Genome 2021; 64(4): 416-25. [http://dx.doi.org/10.1139/gen-2020-0131] [PMID: 33091314]

[28] Mesko B. The role of artificial intelligence in precision medicine. Expert Rev Precis Med Drug Dev 2017; 2(5): 239-41. [http://dx.doi.org/10.1080/23808993.2017.1380516]

[29] Uddin M, Wang Y, Woodbury-Smith M. Artificial intelligence for precision medicine in neurodevelopmental disorders. NPJ Digit Med 2019; 2(1): 112. [http://dx.doi.org/10.1038/s41746-019-0191-0] [PMID: 31799421]

[30] Li L, Zhang W, Tu X, *et al.* Application of Artificial Intelligence in Precision Medicine for Diabetic Macular Edema. Asia Pac J Ophthalmol (Phila) 2023; 12(5): 486-94. [http://dx.doi.org/10.1097/APO.0000000000000583] [PMID: 36650089]

[31] Chen M, Copley SJ, Viola P, Lu H, Aboagye EO. Radiomics and artificial intelligence for precision medicine in lung cancer treatment. Semin Cancer Biol 2023; 93: 97-113. [http://dx.doi.org/10.1016/j.semcancer.2023.05.004] [PMID: 37211292]

[32] Chen PZ, Wang H. [Precision nutrition in the era of precision medicine]. Chin J Prev Med 2016; 50(12): 1036-42. [http://dx.doi.org/10.3760/cma.j.issn.0253-9624.2016.12.004] [PMID: 28057105]

[33] Simpson SJ, Le Couteur DG, James DE, *et al.* The Geometric Framework for Nutrition as a tool in precision medicine. Nutr Healthy Aging 2017; 4(3): 217-26. [http://dx.doi.org/10.3233/NHA-170027] [PMID: 29276791]

[34] Moore JB. From personalised nutrition to precision medicine: The rise of consumer genomics and digital health. Proceedings of the Nutrition Society. [http://dx.doi.org/10.1017/S0029665120006977]

[35] Sawicki C, Haslam D, Bhupathiraju S. Utilising the precision nutrition toolkit in the path towards precision medicine. [http://dx.doi.org/10.1017/S0029665123003038]

[36] Naithani N, Sinha S, Misra P, Vasudevan B, Sahu R. Precision medicine: Concept and tools. Med J Armed Forces India 2021; 77(3): 249-57. [http://dx.doi.org/10.1016/j.mjafi.2021.06.021] [PMID: 34305276]

[37] Woolfenden S, Farrar MA, Eapen V, *et al.* Delivering paediatric precision medicine: Genomic and environmental considerations along the causal pathway of childhood neurodevelopmental disorders.

Dev Med Child Neurol 2022; 64(9): 1077-84.
[http://dx.doi.org/10.1111/dmcn.15289] [PMID: 35661141]

[38] Shojima N, Yamauchi T. Progress in genetics of type 2 diabetes and diabetic complications. J Diabetes Investig 2023; 14(4): 503-15.
[http://dx.doi.org/10.1111/jdi.13970] [PMID: 36639962]

[39] Galiero R, Caturano A, Vetrano E, *et al.* Precision Medicine in Type 2 Diabetes Mellitus: Utility and Limitations. Diabetes Metab Syndr Obes 2023; 16: 3669-89.
[http://dx.doi.org/10.2147/DMSO.S390752] [PMID: 38028995]

[40] Velmovitsky PE, Bevilacqua T, Alencar P, Cowan D, Morita PP. Convergence of Precision Medicine and Public Health Into Precision Public Health: Toward a Big Data Perspective. Front Public Health 2021; 9: 561873.
[http://dx.doi.org/10.3389/fpubh.2021.561873] [PMID: 33889555]

[41] Proper SP, Azouz NP, Mersha TB. Achieving Precision Medicine in Allergic Disease: Progress and Challenges. Front Immunol 2021; 12: 720746.
[http://dx.doi.org/10.3389/fimmu.2021.720746] [PMID: 34484229]

[42] Weerasinghe K, Scahill SL, Pauleen DJ, Taskin N. Big data analytics for clinical decision-making: Understanding health sector perceptions of policy and practice. Technol Forecast Soc Change 2022; 174: 121222.
[http://dx.doi.org/10.1016/j.techfore.2021.121222]

[43] Qoronfleh MW, Chouchane L, Mifsud B, Al Emadi M, Ismail S. THE FUTURE OF MEDICINE, healthcare innovation through precision medicine: policy case study of Qatar. Life Sci Soc Policy 2020; 16(1): 12.
[http://dx.doi.org/10.1186/s40504-020-00107-1] [PMID: 33129349]

[44] AI in Healthcare: Enhancing Diagnosis, Treatment, and Healthcare Systems for a Smarter Future in India. Advances in Bioengineering and Biomedical Science Research 2023; 6(10): 171-7.
[http://dx.doi.org/10.33140/ABBSR.06.10.02]

CHAPTER 3

Unlocking the Power of the Internet of Medical Things: Revolutionizing Healthcare

Prashant Panwar[1,*], **Nekul Chauhan**[2], **Yogita Ambavta**[3] and **Ravikant Dixit**[4]

[1] *KR Mangalam University, India*

[2] *Biomedical Science, London Metropolitan University, London, UK*

[3] *Unity P.G. College, Lucknow, RR Mangalam University, India*

[4] *CPJ College, Uttar Pradesh, India*

Abstract: The Internet of Medical Things (IoMT) revolutionizes healthcare by establishing connections between medical equipment and systems to provide more intelligent and streamlined care. This study examines the transformative influence of the Internet of Medical Things (IoMT) on healthcare, with a specific emphasis on its capacity to improve patient outcomes using remote monitoring, tailored treatment, and the management of chronic diseases. Additionally, it analyses how the Internet of Medical Things (IoMT) improves the effectiveness of healthcare operations, resulting in cost reduction and streamlined workflows. With the increasing adoption of the Internet of Medical Things (IoMT), it is crucial to prioritize strong security and data privacy. This involves implementing effective cybersecurity measures and adhering to regulatory compliance to safeguard patient data. Despite the presence of hurdles such as interoperability and infrastructure needs, the future of the Internet of Medical Things (IoMT) holds the potential for a healthcare system that is more interconnected and efficient. Healthcare providers can achieve better patient care, optimize resource allocation, and contribute to a healthier future by adopting the Internet of Medical Things (IoMT).

Keywords: AI, Automation, Blockchain, Connected devices, Cloud computing, Data analytics, Digital health, IoMT, Interoperability, Predictive analytics, Patient-centric care, Remote monitoring, Smart healthcare, Telemedicine, Wearables.

INTRODUCTION

The Internet of Medical Things (IoMT) represents a revolutionary change in healthcare technology by combining interconnected medical equipment, software

* **Corresponding author Prashant Panwar:** KR Mangalam University, India;
E-mail: Prashantpanwar1565@gmail.com

Neeraj Gupta, Abdelhameed Ibrahim, Bhavesh Vyas & Shobhna Jeet (Eds.)

applications, and healthcare systems into a unified network. This network enables the uninterrupted and smooth data transfer, substantially revolutionizing the provision of medical treatment and clinical procedures. The Internet of Medical Things (IoMT) enables intelligent medical equipment and sensors to monitor and control health issues in real-time, providing a proactive approach to healthcare.

The Internet of Medical Things (IoMT) revolves around interconnected medical equipment, including wearable sensors, remote monitoring tools, and smart implants. These devices collect a vast amount of health data, including vital signs and patient activity levels, and send this information to healthcare providers. The continuous stream of data improves the capacity to monitor health patterns, identify potential problems early, and make more knowledgeable choices regarding medical treatment and care.

In addition, the Internet of Medical Things (IoMT) facilitates a transition towards healthcare guided by data, where immediate observations result in more individualized and effective patient treatment. The incorporation of these devices into Electronic Health Records (EHRs) and other healthcare systems enables enhanced collaboration among healthcare practitioners and enhances overall patient outcomes. The ongoing development of the Internet of Medical Things (IoMT) holds the potential to bring about substantial progress in the delivery and experience of healthcare. This signifies the emergence of a new era characterized by interconnected and intelligent medical technology [1].

THE TRANSFORMATIVE IMPACT OF IOMT ON PATIENT CARE AND OUTCOMES

The Internet of Medical Things (IoMT) has greatly transformed patient care by improving healthcare delivery and management. An outstanding advantage of IoMT is its capacity to enhance patient outcomes by implementing more efficient and prompt therapies. Integrating cutting-edge technology, such as wearable devices and remote monitoring tools, enables IoMT to deliver healthcare practitioners immediate and up-to-date information regarding patients' health status. The continuous stream of information allows for more precise and quicker diagnosis, decreasing the probability of problems and enhancing overall health management.

Remote patient monitoring is essential to the Internet of Medical Things (IoMT), enabling healthcare practitioners to monitor patients' vital signs and health indicators remotely. This feature is especially advantageous for managing chronic illnesses, as it enables ongoing monitoring without regular face-to-face appointments. Regular monitoring and rapid adjustments to treatment programs based on real-time data can benefit patients with diabetes, heart disease, or respiratory disorders. Adopting this proactive strategy aids in properly treating symptoms and mitigating potential health emergencies.

In addition, the Internet of Medical Things (IoMT) allows for the customization of healthcare by adapting treatment strategies to each patient's specific requirements. The comprehensive data gathered from intelligent devices enables a more nuanced comprehension of each patient's well-being, resulting in tailored interventions and more accurate treatment approaches. Personalization increases the efficacy of care and enhances patient pleasure and involvement.

To summarize, the IoMT has a significant and far-reaching effect on patient treatment and results. The Internet of Medical Things (IoMT) is revolutionizing healthcare by utilizing advanced remote monitoring, optimizing the treatment of chronic illnesses, and providing tailored healthcare solutions. This trend is leading to a new era of care that is more impactful, efficient, and focused on the patient's needs [2].

STREAMLINING HEALTHCARE OPERATIONS WITH IOMT: INCREASED EFFICIENCY AND COST SAVINGS

The Internet of Medical Things (IoMT) transforms hospital operations by significantly improving efficiency and decreasing expenses. Healthcare facilities may enhance operational efficiency by integrating interconnected medical equipment and intelligent technology. This integration enables them to streamline processes, make informed decisions based on data analysis, and allocate resources in a more efficient manner.

IoMT significantly enhances healthcare efficiency by optimizing workflows. Integrating devices and systems facilitates effortless communication between many components of the healthcare ecosystem, thereby decreasing reliance on manual data input and mitigating errors. This automation expedites patient registration, data acquisition, and information dissemination, resulting in more streamlined operations and decreased administrative encumbrances.

The Internet of Medical Things (IoMT) also helps to save costs by improving resource allocation. By utilizing real-time data obtained from remote monitoring devices and smart sensors, healthcare providers can better understand patient requirements and effectively allocate resources based on priority. Monitoring equipment can facilitate identifying patients needing rapid attention, hence optimizing the utilization of medical personnel and resources. This focused strategy not only decreases unneeded treatments and hospital admissions but also decreases overall operational expenses.

In addition, the Internet of Medical Things (IoMT) facilitates data-based decision-making by offering healthcare practitioners extensive and up-to-date information. Analyzing the extensive data gathered from interconnected devices can help uncover patterns, and enhance treatment regimens and overall care plans. By adopting an evidence-based approach, therapies' effectiveness is improved, and the chances of expensive errors or unnecessary treatments are reduced.

To summarize, the Internet of Medical Things (IoMT) is essential for optimizing healthcare processes by enhancing productivity and generating financial benefits. The Internet of Medical Things (IoMT) improves the efficiency and cost-effectiveness of the healthcare system by implementing streamlined workflows, allocating resources effectively, and making decisions based on data.

ENSURING ROBUST SECURITY AND DATA PRIVACY IN THE IOMT ECOSYSTEM

With the increasing prevalence of the Internet of Medical Things (IoMT) in healthcare, it is crucial to prioritize strong security measures and protect data privacy. The interconnectivity of IoMT devices gives rise to possible vulnerabilities that necessitate attention to safeguard sensitive patient data and uphold confidence in healthcare technologies.

Data Privacy: Safeguarding patient data is a significant concern within the Internet of Medical Things (IoMT) ecosystem. Healthcare providers must guarantee the confidentiality and authorized use of data obtained by linked devices. Implementing robust encryption techniques and secure data storage protocols protects patient information from illegal access and breaches.

Regulatory Compliance: Complying with regulatory norms is crucial for upholding data privacy and security in the Internet of Medical Things (IoMT). Regulations such as the Health Insurance Portability and Accountability Act (HIPAA) in the United States and the General Data Protection Regulation (GDPR) in Europe provide strict guidelines for managing patient data. Adhering to these requirements guarantees that healthcare businesses fulfill their legal responsibilities and maintain exceptional levels of data security.

Cybersecurity Measures: Strong cybersecurity measures are essential to protect against potential threats in the Internet of Medical Things (IoMT) environment. This involves implementing sophisticated security protocols, such as multi-factor authentication, regular software updates, and intrusion detection systems. Conducting regular security assessments and vulnerability testing is beneficial for identifying and resolving any holes in the system.

Patient Data Protection: To ensure the safeguarding of patient data, it is necessary to implement both technological measures and develop explicit policies and processes for data management. Providing healthcare professionals with instruction on the most effective methods for safeguarding data and promoting a mindset of constant awareness can significantly strengthen the safeguarding of confidential information [3].

OVERCOMING CHALLENGES AND EMBRACING THE FUTURE OF IOMT IN HEALTHCARE

The use of the Internet of Medical Things (IoMT) in healthcare has the potential to bring about significant transformation. However, various problems must be overcome to realize its full benefits. A considerable challenge is integrating IoMT technologies into current healthcare systems. A significant challenge faced by numerous healthcare facilities is the presence of antiquated infrastructure and the reluctance of staff members to embrace change. For successful adoption, it is essential to ensure that new Internet of Medical Things (IoMT) devices and systems can easily fit into existing processes and practices. This includes making both technological and cultural adaptations within businesses [4].

Interoperability presents a significant obstacle. The healthcare industry employs various devices from multiple manufacturers, each according to distinct standards and norms. For the Internet of Medical Things (IoMT) to be efficient, these devices must possess the capability to exchange and transmit data regularly. Establishing and following universal standards and protocols is crucial for resolving interoperability challenges and guaranteeing seamless collaboration among IoMT systems.

The presence of infrastructure requirements also presents a substantial obstacle. Deploying IoMT solutions typically requires significant investment in infrastructure, such as high-speed internet, secure data storage, and powerful analytics capabilities. Healthcare organizations must anticipate and make arrangements for the financial and technical requirements associated with supporting these technologies. This entails allocating resources to develop and maintain strong systems and ensuring that people possess the requisite technical proficiency to manage and sustain them effectively [5].

The revolution in the healthcare sector, propelled by the Internet of Medical Things (IoMT), encompasses not only technological advancements but also necessitates alterations in organizational culture and procedures. Healthcare personnel must undergo continuous education and training to adapt to new care delivery methods, such as remote monitoring and data-driven decision-making.

To fully capitalize on the advantages of IoMT, embracing the changes that occur as the sector progresses is crucial.

In the coming years, several developments are expected to impact the direction of IoMT significantly. The progress in artificial intelligence and machine learning is anticipated to improve the functionalities of IoMT devices, resulting in more precise diagnosis and customized treatment alternatives. Furthermore, the proliferation of 5G technology is expected to enhance the connectivity and efficiency of Internet of Medical Things (IoMT) devices, enabling more effective real-time data transmission. To fully leverage the potential of IoMT and achieve significant enhancements in patient care and healthcare delivery, healthcare organizations must proactively anticipate and adapt to emerging trends and breakthroughs [6].

CONCLUSION: EMBRACING THE IOMT REVOLUTION FOR A HEALTHIER, MORE CONNECTED FUTURE

Utilizing the potential of the Internet of Medical Things (IoMT) offers a crucial chance for healthcare professionals to transform care delivery. Healthcare organizations can enhance care provision by implementing Internet of Medical Things (IoMT) technologies, which deliver personalized, efficient, and cost-effective healthcare services. The Internet of Medical Things (IoMT) enables continuous real-time monitoring and data collection, enabling more accurate and prompt actions. This not only improves patient outcomes but also optimizes the use of resources, decreasing operational costs and enhancing overall healthcare efficiency.

Incorporating the Internet of Medical Things (IoMT) into healthcare systems effectively tackles numerous critical difficulties the sector faces. By continuously monitoring and analyzing health data, healthcare providers may make well-informed judgments and customize therapies to meet each patient's specific needs. The adoption of data-driven care results in improved treatment of chronic diseases, enhanced effectiveness of preventive interventions, and a superior level of patient care. Moreover, the potential of the Internet of Medical Things (IoMT) to optimize workflows and promote seamless communication between devices and systems holds the promise of enhancing the effectiveness of healthcare delivery.

Adopting this technological revolution is crucial for maintaining competitiveness in a progressively intricate healthcare environment. Implementing the Internet of Medical Things (IoMT) necessitates financial investment in technology and a dedication to addressing infrastructure, interoperability, and regulatory compliance obstacles. To become pioneers in the future of healthcare, healthcare institutions must confront these difficulties directly and cultivate a culture of innovation.

Now is the opportune moment to begin the voyage into the realm of the Internet of Medical Things (IoMT). Healthcare professionals may lead the way towards a future that is more interconnected, streamlined, and focused on the needs of patients by embracing and incorporating this cutting-edge technology. Join the Internet of Medical Things (IoMT) revolution now to bring about significant changes in healthcare and contribute to a better society for everyone [7].

REFERENCES

[1] Riazul Islam SM, Daehan Kwak , Humaun Kabir M, Hossain M, Kyung-Sup Kwak . The internet of things for health care: A comprehensive survey. IEEE Access 2015; 3: 678-708. [http://dx.doi.org/10.1109/ACCESS.2015.2437951]

[2] Albahri AS, Hamid RA, Alwan JK, *et al.* Role of Internet of Medical Things (IoMT) in COVID-19 pandemic: Current trends and future perspectives. J Med Syst 2020; 44(7): 122. [http://dx.doi.org/10.1007/s10916-020-01582-x] [PMID: 32451808]

[3] Mendez AJ, Gonzalez LA, López-Vallejo M, *et al.* Security and privacy in IoMT: Challenges and solutions. Sensors (Basel) 2020; 20(20): 5893. [PMID: 33080979]

[4] Yang P, Dai L, Zheng Q, *et al.* Enhancing healthcare outcomes with IoMT-enabled remote monitoring systems: Opportunities and challenges. IEEE Rev Biomed Eng 2023; 16: 145-63.

[5] Roco MC, Bainbridge WS. Converging technologies for improving human performance: Nanotechnology, biotechnology, information technology and cognitive science. Res Technol Manag 2003. [http://dx.doi.org/10.1007/978-94-017-0359-8]

[6] [6]. Al-Joboury M, Hemiary EH. Internet of Things Architecture Based Cloud for Healthcare. Iraqi Journal of Information & Communications Technology. 2018. [http://dx.doi.org/10.31987/ijict.1.1.7]

[7] Zhou B. A wireless internet of things architecture based on mobile internet. Int J Online Eng. 2017. [http://dx.doi.org/10.3991/ijoe.v13i10.7745]

CHAPTER 4

Comparative Analysis of IoMT-based Lung Disease Classification using Deep Learning in Healthcare

Garima Verma[1,*] and **Shiva Prakash**[2]

[1] *Department of Cyber Security, School of Computer Science and Engineering, Galgotias University, Greater Noida, Uttar Pradesh, India*

[2] *Department of ITCA, Madan Mohan Malaviya University of Technology, Gorakhpur, India*

Abstract: Lung diseases cover a wide range of conditions that affect how we breathe and create serious public health issues. This chapter gives an organized overview of pulmonary disorders, sorting them by anatomical areas and disease features. A thorough review of recent literature shows new progress in finding and classifying lung diseases, mainly focusing on computer-based methods. The chapter also examines the role of deep learning, a component of artificial intelligence, in addressing complex diagnostic tasks that have traditionally relied on human expertise. By utilizing neural networks and data-driven methods, deep learning enables the accurate identification of lung infections and enhances predictions in clinical settings. The chapter discusses new technologies like machine learning, the Internet of Things (IoT), and intelligent sensing systems for their potential to change respiratory healthcare. The aim is to update researchers and practitioners on the convergence of biomedical science and innovative computing.

Keywords: CNN Model, Challenges, Deep learning, IoMT (Internet of Medical Things), Lung diseases.

INTRODUCTION

The Internet of Medical Things (IoMT) is nowadays connecting many devices and wearables all over the world for the quick processing of data. Notably, occupational exposures have demonstrated relevance in contexts such as tuberculosis and the recent COVID-19 pandemic [1]. Lung cancer is a disease caused by the abnormal development of cells. Other environmental factors connected to lung infection include asbestos, radon gas, air contamination, and synthetic compounds like uranium, beryllium, vinyl chloride, and arsenic [2]. These conditions may vary, ranging from a bit of discomfort to critical situations.

* **Corresponding author Garima Verma:** Department of Cyber Security, School of Computer Science and Engineering, Galgotias University, Greater Noida, Uttar Pradesh, India; E-mail: garimaverma311016@gmail.com

Neeraj Gupta, Abdelhameed Ibrahim, Bhavesh Vyas & Shobhna Jeet (Eds.)

The findings revealed that higher cumulative cigarette usage correlated with diminished lung function, increased likelihood of respiratory symptoms, and a potential connection to instances of COPD within the HIV-positive group [3]. Air pollution is the mixture of all toxic gases and particles. These gaseous particles disseminate deep into our lungs and cause serious respiratory problems [4].

Infections, environmental factors, genetic predispositions, or a combination of these factors mainly cause lung diseases. The outcomes, particularly for non-smoker individuals, accentuate a direct and meaningful connection between antecedent lung diseases and the probability of developing lung cancer [5]. They can affect anyone, regardless of age or gender [6]. It consists of a series of tubes and passages that allow air to enter and exit the lungs. Neural networks enable them to learn and represent complex patterns in data. Pneumonia is an infection affecting the lungs, leading to the accumulation of infected fluid in the alveoli of one or both lungs, causing breathing-related difficulties [7]. Different symptoms of lung infections are chest pain, breathing problems, cough, fever, and fatigue. There is community-acquired pneumonia, which continues to be a significant contributor to both illness and mortality [8]. Fig. (**1**) illustrates a clear chest X-ray image of a patient with asthma.

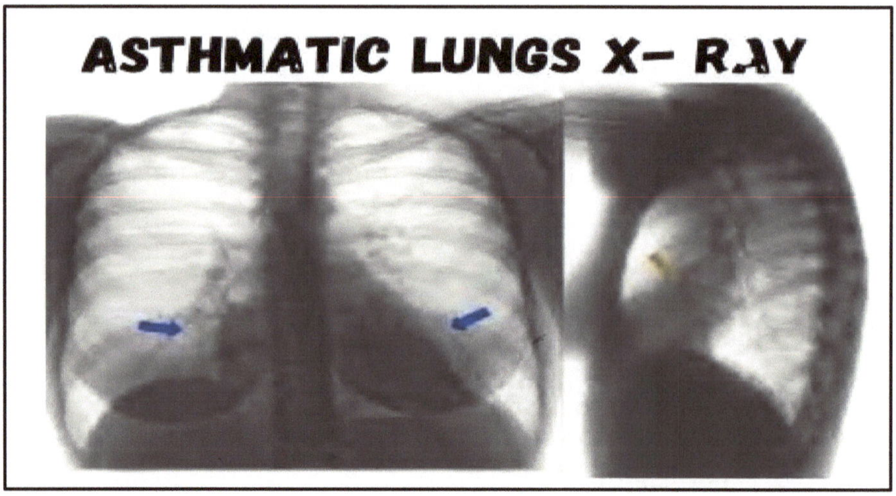

Fig. (1). Lung X-ray [8].

In the realm of pneumonia detection, many studies have incorporated TL approaches and data augmentation techniques. For instance, Tobias et al. have directly employed Convolutional Neural Networks (CNNs) [9]. In contrast, Stephen et al. have trained the CNN model from scratch, and also applied different augmentation techniques like scaling, rotation, zooming, height shift, shear, and flipping [10]. Several other authors [11 - 13] have opted for pre-trained CNNs to detect pneumonia. Notably, some studies also introduced data augmentation techniques to enhance the training mechanisms in training datasets, for instance, Rajpurkar et al. have used horizontal flipping [14] for pneumonia detection. At the same time, Ayan and Ünver [15] have utilized convolutional networks to detect pneumonia. Recent studies have demonstrated the effectiveness of transfer learning and convolutional neural networks in diagnosing pneumonia from chest X-ray images [16, 17], highlighting both the promise and challenges of deploying such models in clinical settings. Respiratory diseases such as asthma and COPD are characterized by airway obstruction or narrowing, which reduces airflow and impairs breathing. Relative Risk (RR) is the most common metric used in epidemiology to compare the likelihood of developing a respiratory condition. When amalgamated, the cumulative risk stemming from these conditions yielded an overarching relative risk of 1.80.

Furthermore, individuals with prior bouts of pneumonia exhibited a lung cancer risk of 1.43, while those with a tuberculosis history carried a risk of 1.76. Despite a reduction in the observed effect among non-smokers, the risk remained appreciable for both pneumonia (RR = 1.36) and tuberculosis (RR = 1.90). Table **1** summarizes the CNN frameworks specifying the datasets that various authors have used in recent years.

Table 1. Comparative analysis of different deep learning frameworks.

Deep learning techniques	Dataset	references
Deep Siamese-based neural network	Unspecified Kaggle dataset	[18]
Use of augmentation and TL	LDOCTCXR	[19]
CNN with a majority voting technique	LDOCTCXR	[12]
CNN with transfer learning	LDOCTCXR	[20]
CNN, along with an LSTM model	Mooney Dataset	[21]
Use of CNN for lung disease detection	2018 RSNA dataset	[22]
CNN, along with a hybrid technique	NIH Dataset	[23]
CNN with TL	Private dataset	[24]

According to the latest statement of the World Health Organization (WHO), tuberculosis is one of the most critical causes of death in the world [25, 26]. One approach, demonstrated by Heo et al. [27], involves utilizing social factors, including height, weight, and age, to enhance the overall performance of the CNN model. Table **2** shows the comparative study of different deep learning techniques.

Table 2. Comparative analysis of different deep learning techniques and datasets.

DL Techniques	Datasets	Authors
Convolutional Neural Network	Used Private dataset	[28]
ViDi	Unspecified	[29]
KNN algorithm, Linear Regression, and Sequential Minimal Optimization Classification	Shenzhen	[30]
CNN + Transfer Learning + data augmentation	Montgomery	[31]
CNN technique	Image CLEF dataset of 2018	[32]
CNN + Transfer Learning + demographic Information	Private dataset	[33]
CNN + Data Augmentation + Ensemble Method	Montgomery	[34]
CNN + Transfer Learning + Data augmentation	Private dataset	[35]
Modified maximum pattern margin support vector machine	Private datasets	[36]
CAD4TB + clinical information	Private datasets	[37]
DBN	Ziehl Neelsen Sputum	[38]
Neural network	Montgomery, Shenzhen	[39]

A prominent cause of lung cancer involves the presence of pulmonary nodules, which are in the form of compact tissue structures that become visible within the lungs and their surrounding areas [40]. These nodules are discernible through CT scan images and may exhibit either malignancy, indicating a cancerous nature, or benignity, signifying a non-cancerous state [41]. It is essential to comprehend the various factors that contribute to lung disease.

- Infections: bacteria, viruses, and fungi can infect the lungs, leading to conditions like pneumonia, tuberculosis, and fungal lung infections.
- Irritants: very long exposure to heavy irritants may lead to lung-related critical problems.
- Allergies: allergic reactions can trigger conditions like asthma, where the airways become inflamed and constricted, causing breathing difficulties.
- Genetic factors: Certain lung diseases, such as cystic fibrosis, are caused by genetic mutations that affect the production of mucus, leading to lung infections.
- Autoimmune disorders: Certain autoimmune diseases can cause the immune system to mistakenly attack lung tissue, resulting in conditions like rheumatoid arthritis-associated interstitial lung disease.

- Environmental factors: exposure to environmental hazards, such as asbestos and silica dust, can lead to lung diseases.

The Internet of Medical Things (IoMT) plays a crucial role in data collection and processing in healthcare domains [42]. IoMT allows for the easy collection and storage of data at specified locations, such as in the cloud. The data can be processed using various machine learning techniques for further analysis and interpretation. Respiratory illnesses are one of the leading causes of global fatalities, as discussed in this paper [43].

A significant portion of the population consistently experiences various forms of lung function disorders, which ultimately pave the way for respiratory ailments [44, 45]. Vital actions in managing these conditions include prevention and the prompt identification of symptoms. To mitigate mortality rates, the development of a practical detection framework becomes imperative.

ANATOMICAL AND CLINICAL PERSPECTIVES ON LUNG DISEASES

This section examines the primary causes of lung disease and outlines current treatment strategies and potential solutions. A notable hurdle encountered during this research revolved around sourcing accessible data from the public domain and subsequently rectifying inaccurately documented records [46]. Due to the limited availability of respiratory datasets, numerous studies have emerged focusing on the detection and classification of respiratory diseases. Each of these works introduces distinct predictive models, often leveraging advanced deep learning techniques, as highlighted in this paper [47].

- **Various Applications used in Deep Learning and Biomedicine**

In a part of the series "Studies of Big Data" (volume 68), "deep learning techniques for Biomedical and Health Informatics," Mittal [51] has provided various insights and developments into artificial neural networks and also discussed their applications. Biomedical engineering is one of the emerging interdisciplinary domains that combine information science, computer science, and healthcare [48]. It leverages deep learning techniques to efficiently analyze vast amounts of healthcare data, including patient records, with the goal of improving healthcare quality and patient outcomes. The article addresses the lack of comprehensive resources in this emerging and rapidly evolving field, providing insights into the latest research methodologies, developments, case studies, and trends. It aims to facilitate the work of both new and experienced researchers, ultimately contributing to the betterment of human life and healthcare through the understanding of deep learning models [49]. Neural networks help represent medical concepts from existing electronic health records, enabling analysis and prediction [50]. They realized that deep learning can perform better in classical analysis, varied datasets, and machine classification methods. They also explained the applications of various deep learning algorithms used in physiological disease detection [51].

Building upon these foundational insights, this chapter provides a concise overview of the applications of deep learning in healthcare. It focuses on the analysis of biomedical images, both electrical and non-electrical biomedical signals, and fundamental concepts related to Electrocardiograms (ECG), as well as relevant databases. The discussion highlights how deep learning techniques can enhance the understanding and interpretation of these various types of biomedical data. Moreover, the issues in producing ECG and the near future of deep learning in healthcare are also described [52]. While some studies achieved promising accuracies, challenges such as noise removal, data normalization, and the limited scope of datasets affected their results. Some models focus on specific respiratory issues, such as wheeze or pneumonia, while others classify a range of pulmonary diseases. Despite advancements, limitations exist in terms of overall accuracy, comprehensiveness, and potential for wider disease classification. Researchers [45] developed an approach for classifying lung diseases using a publicly accessible dataset. They applied data normalization techniques to recalibrate audio samples, bolstering accuracy. Their work yielded a novel lung disease classification (IDC) system, incorporating various normalization and augmentation strategies, albeit adding complexity due to its unique approach to IDC. Notably, the project focuses solely on classifying wheezes and everyday sounds, omitting recognition of other abnormal respiratory sounds or diseases.

The respiratory airway refers to the series of passages and structures through which air travels as it enters and exits the lungs during the process of breathing. It encompasses both the upper and lower respiratory tracts, each with distinct functions and anatomical characteristics. Diseases that can affect these airways are given below:

- **Asthma disease**

Asthma is a major chronic respiratory problem that affects the air passages in the lungs, making it difficult for individuals to breathe. It is mainly caused by inflammation of the air passage, which triggers the critical condition of the patient. These factors can increase the chances of asthma in genetically susceptible individuals. Some of the common environmental factors and triggers associated with the development of asthma include environmental factors such as air pollutants, vehicle exhaust, and industrial emissions have been associated with the development and exacerbation of asthma. Allergens, respiratory infections, and tobacco smoke are also problems caused by air pollution. Respiratory infections caused by viruses, particularly during early childhood, have been linked to an increased risk of developing asthma.

- **COPD (Chronic Obstructive Pulmonary Disease)**

COPD is a critical chronic lung disease that primarily affects the air passages and makes breathing difficult. It is often characterized by persistent airflow limitation, which is not fully reversible. Fig. (**2**) represents the systematic structure and significant parts of COPD (Chronic Obstructive Pulmonary Disease). The two main conditions that fall under the umbrella term COPD are bronchitis and emphysema.

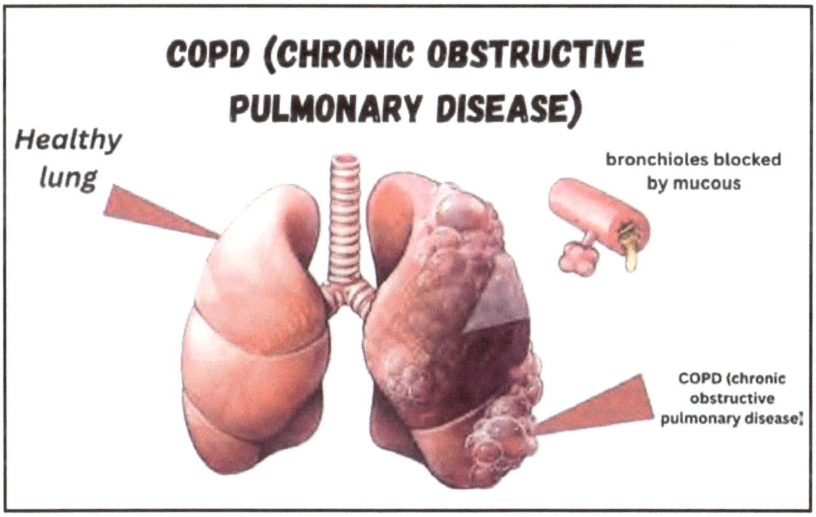

Fig. (2). Systematic Structure of COPD [53].

Numerous studies in the literature have employed Convolutional Neural Networks (CNNs) for the classification of tuberculosis. The conclusion drawn from these studies shows high values for the Area Under the Receiver Operating Characteristic Curve (AUC), along with high sensitivity values, and the overall performance has significantly improved for the Chest X-ray dataset.

Furthermore, additional studies demonstrate improved classification for various diseases, including tuberculosis, skin disease, and cancer classification, which utilize the latest approaches such as transfer learning and ensemble methods.

• Lung Cancer

Lung cancer is a critical problem that originates from the abnormal division of cells in the lungs. When these cells undergo significant changes that result in irregular growth, it leads to the formation of tumors. It is a complex and severe disease with different types and stages, each requiring specific approaches to diagnosis and treatment.

Lung cancer's association with smoking was recognized in the mid-20th century. Before this, the link between lung cancer and tobacco use was not well understood. During the tenure from 1950 to 1960, research started to establish a strong correlation between smoking and lung cancer, leading to public health campaigns to raise awareness about the dangers of smoking. These efforts contributed to decreased smoking rates in some parts of the world, but lung cancer remains a significant health issue due to the prolonged latency period between smoking and cancer development. Fig. (**3**) represents the diagrammatic structure of Pulmonary Edema. Detection of lung cancer using deep learning is discussed in the papers cited.

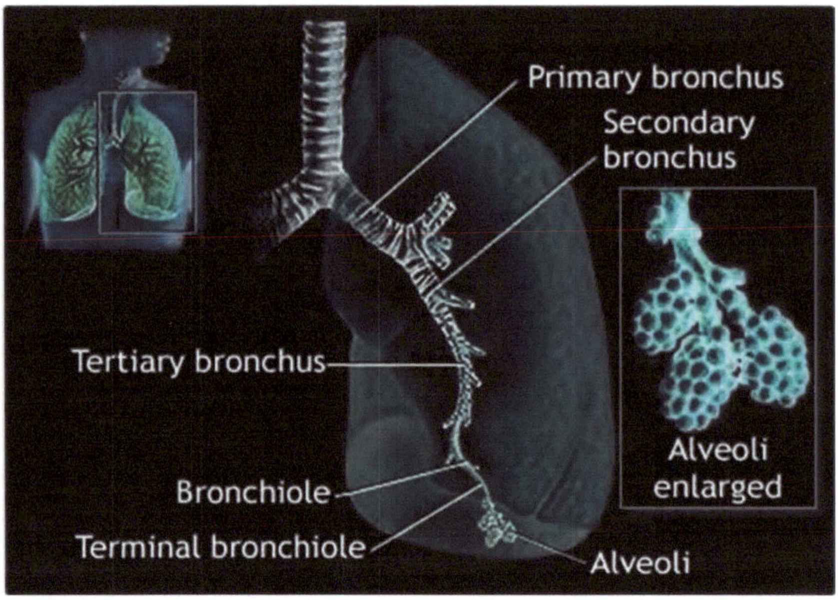

Fig. (3). Structure of pulmonary edema [54].

- **Acute respiratory distress syndrome (ARDS)**

This problem occurs when there is a significant inflammation that causes heavy damage to the small air sacs (alveoli), which leads to fluid buildup, impaired oxygen exchange, and difficulty breathing.

ARDS can result from various underlying conditions and can lead to low oxygen levels in the bloodstream, organ dysfunction, and even death if not treated promptly. ARDS requires intensive care management, and treatment often takes place in an Intensive Care Unit (ICU).

While many patients recover, the severity of the condition can lead to long-term lung damage in some cases. Fig. (**4**) shows a clear distinction between normal lungs and cancerous lungs. Preventing ARDS involves addressing its potential triggers, such as prompt treatment of infections and avoiding harmful inhalation of substances.

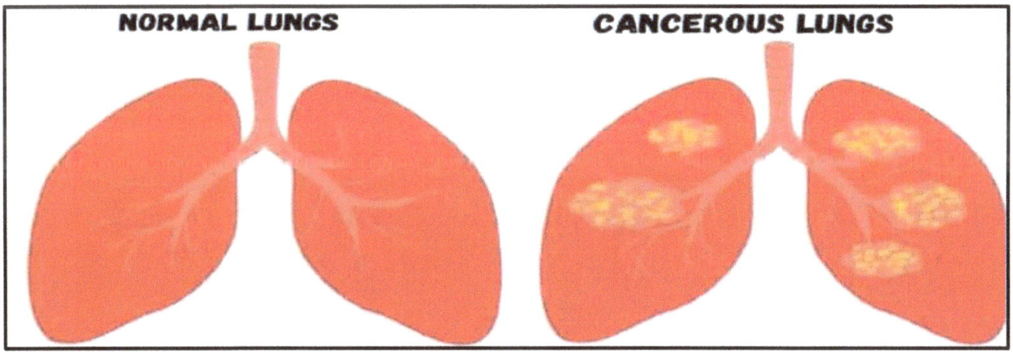

Fig. (4). Normal *vs* cancerous lungs [55].

- **Effect of Lung Diseases on the Interstitium**

It is a complex network of tissues found within the body, particularly in organs such as the lungs, skin, and digestive tract. The disease affects connective tissues that provide structural support and facilitate the transportation of fluids, gases, and other substances between cells and blood vessels. Fig. (**5**) shows normal alveoli and abnormal alveoli in the interstitium-based lung disease framework.

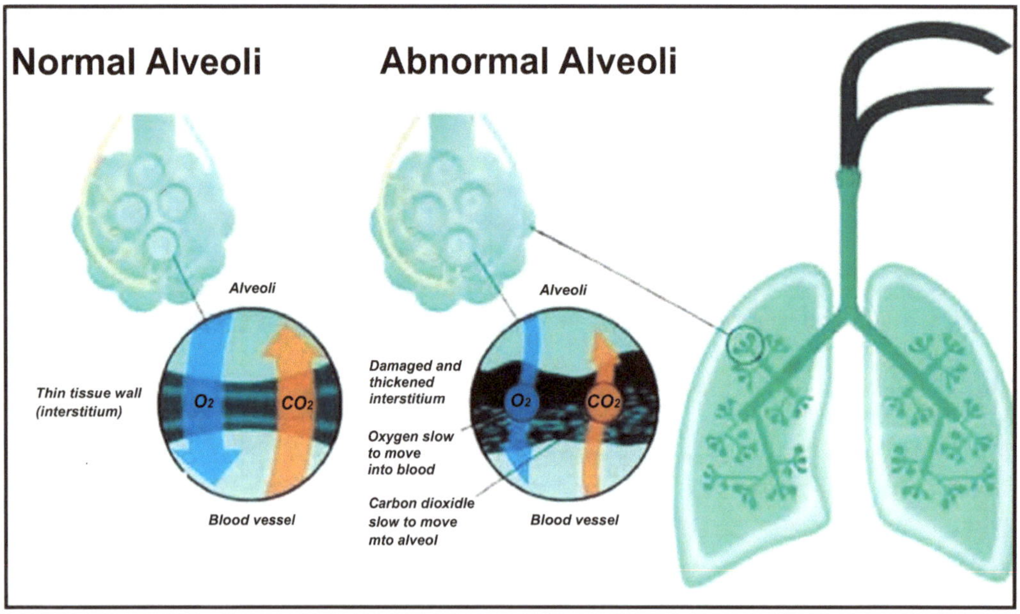

Fig. (5). Interstitium-based lung disease framework [56].

• Effect of Lung Diseases on Blood Vessels

Several lung diseases specifically affect blood vessels within the lungs. These conditions can lead to impaired blood flow, reduced oxygen exchange, and other complications. Here are a few examples of lung diseases that affect blood vessels.

- Pulmonary hypertension (PH): Pulmonary hypertension is a critical scenario characterized by high blood pressure in the pulmonary arteries, which carry blood. PH can result from various underlying causes, including idiopathic (unknown), connective tissue diseases, congenital heart defects, and chronic lung diseases. Treatment aims to manage symptoms.
- Pulmonary embolism (PE): This is a critical issue that occurs when a blood clot forms and then travels from the lungs to the pulmonary artery, blocking the region and leading to decreased blood flow and oxygen exchange, which can cause various issues, including fatigue, chest pain, and shortness of breath.
- Pulmonary venous thromboembolism (PVTE): similar to PE, PVTE involves the formation of blood clots in the veins that drain blood from the lungs. It causes symptoms such as shortness of breath, fatigue, chest pain, and coughing up blood. Treatment involves anticoagulation therapy and addressing underlying causes.

- Idiopathic pulmonary hemosiderosis (IPH): IPH is a rare disorder caused by recurrent bleeding into the lungs, resulting in the accumulation of iron-containing pigment (hemosiderin) within lung tissue. This can lead to iron buildup and damage in the lungs' blood vessels. It often presents with cough, difficulty breathing, and anemia.

- **Effect of Lung diseases on the Pleura**

It plays a significant role in facilitating the smooth movement of the lungs during breathing. Different types of lung diseases can affect the pleura, leading to a range of symptoms and complications. Here are a few examples:

- Pleurisy (pleuritis): Pleurisy is inflammation of the pleura, often caused by infections such as viral or bacterial pneumonia. It can result in sharp chest pain that worsens with breathing or coughing. Pleurisy can also be caused by other conditions like autoimmune diseases (rheumatoid arthritis, lupus) or pulmonary embolism.
- Pleural effusion: This condition is caused by several types of diseases, including infections, heart failure, cancer, and liver disease. Symptoms may include shortness of breath, coughing, and chest discomfort.
- Pneumothorax: It can result from trauma, underlying lung diseases (like emphysema), or occur spontaneously. Various types of symptoms are caused, such as fatigue, sharp chest pain, breathing problems, and rapid heart rate.
- Empyema: Empyema is a complication of bacterial pneumonia in which pus accumulates in the pleural space. It can cause symptoms similar to those of pleurisy or pleural effusion, accompanied by fever and general malaise.
- Pleural tumors: Tumors that originate in the pleura (primary pleural tumors) or spread to the pleura from other sites (secondary pleural tumors) can cause chest pain, difficulty breathing, and other symptoms. Diagnosis and treatment of pleural-related lung diseases depend on the specific condition and its underlying cause.

Medical professionals utilize various types of datasets, including chest X-rays, CT scans, and occasionally procedures such as thoracentesis (fluid removal) or pleural biopsy, to facilitate accurate diagnosis. Treatment strategies vary and may include addressing the underlying cause, draining fluid, managing pain and symptoms, and, in cases of cancer, applying appropriate oncological treatments. Early diagnosis and prompt medical attention are crucial for improving outcomes in pleura-related lung diseases.

• Lung Diseases' Effect on the Chest Wall

Various factors can also affect the chest wall, which consists of various structures, including muscles, bones, and connective tissues that enclose and protect the thoracic cavity. Here are a few examples of lung diseases that can impact the chest wall.

- Kyphoscoliosis: Kyphoscoliosis is a critical condition characterized by distortion in both the lateral (scoliosis) and posterior (kyphosis) directions. Severe curvature can significantly impact lung expansion, leading to reduced lung function and potentially resulting in breathing difficulties.
- Ankylosing spondylitis: This is a kind of inflammatory disease that can lead to fusion of spinal vertebrae. This fusion can limit chest wall mobility, affecting lung function and leading to restrictive lung diseases.
- Muscular dystrophy: Some forms of muscular dystrophy affect the muscles involved in breathing, leading to weakness of the respiratory muscles and reducing the ability to expand the chest during inhalation effectively.
- Rib fractures: Fractured ribs, often caused by trauma, can cause pain and limit chest wall movement. This can affect lung expansion and lead to shallow breathing, potentially increasing the risk of pneumonia.

Treatment approaches for lung diseases affecting the chest wall depend on the specific condition and its underlying cause. Management may involve pain relief, physical therapy to maintain or improve chest wall mobility, and addressing any underlying diseases that contribute to the chest wall-related issues. In some cases, surgical interventions might be considered to address severe deformities or fractures.

PNEUMONIA DETECTION USING DEEP LEARNING TECHNIQUES

The history of deep learning is characterized by periods of innovation, stagnation, and revival. Advancements in neural network architectures, training algorithms, and computing power have driven the field's progression. This section explores the concept of neural networks, explaining their components and providing a mathematical example to illustrate their inputs and outputs.

Artificial Intelligence is the broad domain that comprises a neural network model where a considerable number of nodes are interconnected, recognizing patterns and relationships within the information they are given. Neural networks can learn directly from data, enabling them to uncover hidden patterns more effectively and thereby enhance their overall performance. This feature of adaptability makes neural networks more prominent for use in fields like image classification, voice recognition, language processing, *etc.*

Components of a Neural Network

Neural networks function in a manner similar to how the human brain actually works. Therefore, a neural network consists of several layers as discussed below:

Input layer: This initial layer takes in the raw input from the dataset, performs the necessary mathematical operations, and then forwards the processed information to the hidden layer. For example, for any image-related task, the input values will be in the form of pixels.

Hidden layers: These are the layers where the actual computation and learning take place. This layer processes the input using some mathematical function and forwards the output to the next layer or output layer. Each layer performs its functions and tasks according to its complexity and design.

Output layer: This is the final layer at which data is obtained in the form of classification. In image recognition, this corresponds to the label assigned to the recognized object.

Fig. (**6**) illustrates the basic neural network architecture for deep learning data prediction and classification.

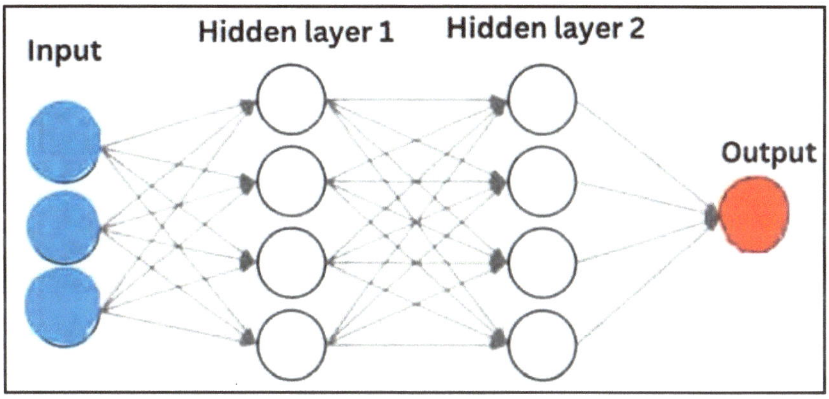

Fig. (6). Deep learning architecture [35]

Mathematical Operations

To elucidate the computational flow within a basic feedforward neural network, consider a single-input, single-output architecture comprising one hidden layer.

Let the input variable be denoted by x, representing a generic feature (*e.g.*, physical measurement, behavioral metric, or environmental parameter), and let the output variable y represent the predicted response.

The network consists of an input layer that receives input x. A hidden layer with weight w_1 and bias b_1 follows. An output layer has weight w_2 and a bias b_2. Each layer applies a nonlinear activation function to introduce representational flexibility. The forward pass proceeds as follows:

The input vector x is transformed linearly and then passed through an activation function

f(.):h = f(w_1 x + b_1).

The hidden representation h undergoes a transformation using another activation function

$g(\cdot)$: $y = g(w_2 h + b_2)$.

This formulation captures the essence of hierarchical feature extraction, where the hidden layer serves as an intermediate representation space. The choice of activation functions f and g (*e.g.*, sigmoid, ReLU, or linear) depends on the nature of the task—classification, regression, or hybrid modeling.

Training the Neural Network

For neural network training, we need a labeled dataset of house sizes and their corresponding prices. The network starts with random weights and iteratively adjusts them using a process called backpropagation. One crucial distinction among neural networks is either they are linear or nonlinear. This classification is based on the types of transformations that neurons apply to their inputs. Let us delve into the concepts of linear and nonlinear neural networks and explore their differences.

Linear Neural Networks

Linear neural networks generally refer to a neural network in which a linear combination of inputs is used to generate outputs, which are further calculated using any activation function. In mathematical terms, a linear combination refers to the process of obtaining the production by summing weighted inputs. Fig. (**7**) shows a single-layer network having inputs and weights in a neural network.

Output = (w1 * input1) + (w2 * input2) + ... +b

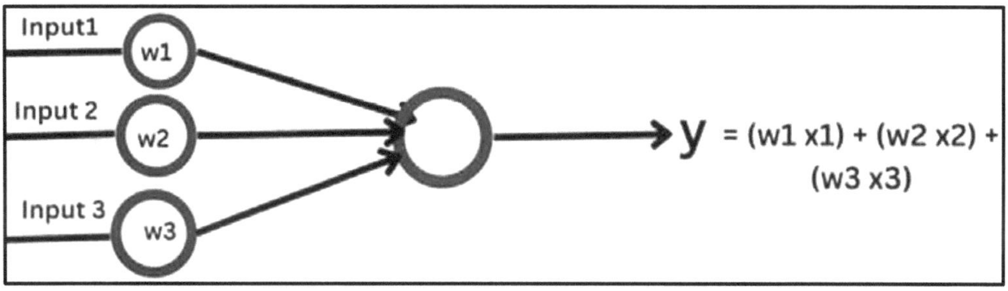

Fig. (7). Single-layer neural network [35].

Here, "w1," "w2," etc., represent the weights associated with each set of input, and "b" denotes the bias term for any prediction value. The activation function applied to the linear combination is usually a simple identity function, which means the output remains linear even after the activation.

Limitations of linear neural networks: Linear neural networks have their limitations. Since their outputs are a cluster of linear combinations of different inputs, they represent a model in the form of linear relationships within data. This restriction makes them ineffective at capturing complex patterns and nonlinear relationships present in many real-world datasets. For instance, linear models would struggle to recognize curved patterns in data or to solve tasks that involve intricate interactions among variables.

Nonlinear Neural Networks

Nonlinear neural networks use various types of activation functions to introduce non-linearity into the network easily. This type of non-linearity helps in mapping and approximating complex computations present in the input dataset. When different nonlinear layers are stacked together, the network achieves the capability of capturing complex patterns, making these networks suitable for various tasks, such as text recognition and image recognition.

Activation functions and non-linearity

Activation functions are used to introduce non-linearity by transforming the weighted input in a nonlinear way. Common activation functions include:

- Rectified linear unit (ReLU): This is one of the most commonly used activation functions, which returns the input as positive or zero values. Mathematically: f(x) = max (0, x). RELU incorporates non-linearity by turning off certain neurons for negative inputs.

- Sigmoid: the sigmoid activation function is an S-shaped graph in which the input lies between 0 and 1, which helps map input values to probabilities.

f(x) = 1 / (1 + exp(-x)) (1)

Hyperbolic tangent (tanh): This activation function is similar to the sigmoidal function, where tanh values range between -1 and 1.

f(y) =(exp(y) - exp(-y)) / (exp(y) + exp(-y)) (2)

Softmax: The SoftMax activation function is often used for multi-class classification in complex networks, which converts a series of vectors of raw scores into a respective probability distribution. It is suitable for problems with multiple possible outcomes.

Advantages of nonlinear neural networks: Nonlinear neural networks can learn complex relationships in data. They can understand complex and hidden patterns and spatial hierarchies, and extract meaningful features from raw data, ultimately leading to improved performance in tasks that involve intricate data structures. In summary, the distinction between linear and nonlinear neural networks lies in the type of activation functions used. Linear neural networks are limited to modeling linear relationships, while nonlinear neural networks use nonlinear activations to capture hidden patterns.

Techniques used in Deep Learning Models

Deep learning neural networks generally use an artificial learning approach to solve a particular task of classification or regression. Various types of architectures and models are used to develop deep learning classifiers, as discussed in Fig. (**8**), which perform some specific tasks according to the requirement. Some prominent types of deep learning approaches have been discussed below:

CONVOLUTIONAL NEURAL NETWORKS

Modern CNN architectures often include various design elements to enhance performance, such as skip connections (*e.g.*, ResNet), attention mechanisms (*e.g.*, transformer-based architectures), and more. The working of CNN is explained below:

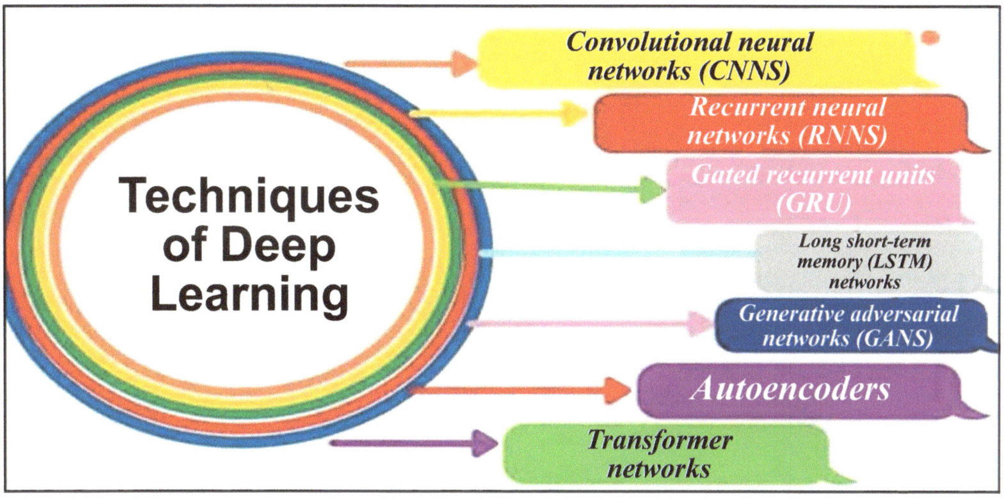

Fig. (8). Types of deep learning models [42].

- **Preprocessing Layer**: In Convolutional Neural Networks (CNNs), there is no specific "preprocessing layer" in the traditional sense, as CNNs are typically designed to extract features directly from the raw data, such as various types of images. However, preprocessing can be an essential part of preparing the data for CNN training. These preprocessing steps are usually performed outside the neural network architecture but are crucial to ensure the network's effectiveness. Some common preprocessing steps for CNNs are:
  - Resizing and Normalization: The images taken from the dataset are often resized to a constant size, ensuring even dimensions, which can be used as input to the CNN. Normalization is applied to different pixel values ranging from 0 to 1 and -1 to +1, which helps the network converge faster during training.
  - Data Augmentation: Various data augmentation techniques, such as horizontal flipping, zooming, and cropping, are applied to create variations in the original images of the dataset. This helps the model become more robust to different viewpoints and orientations.
  - Gray Scaling (Optional): In some cases, color images might be converted to grayscale if color information is not relevant for the task. This reduces the input's dimensionality and computational requirements.
  - Noise Reduction (Optional): Various denoising or noise reduction techniques can be employed, such as Gaussian filters or filtering, to clean up the training dataset.

- Label Encoding and One-Hot Encoding: For classification tasks, labels or class categories are often encoded in numerical form (label encoding) and sometimes further converted into a binary vector. Fig. (**9**) represents a CNN architecture with feature extraction and the classification phase.
- Pooling layer: This layer helps reduce the dimension of the input training dataset by representing a feature map corresponding to each input, while retaining the necessary information. There are three types of pooling techniques used at this particular layer:
  - Max pool
  - Min pool
  - Average pool
- Fully connected layers: This layer utilizes the flattened input images and leverages key features to make further predictions. This is the most responsible layer for classification-related tasks.
- Output layer: This is the final layer where the output is obtained in the form of classification or regression. For image classification, this might involve SoftMax activation to produce class probabilities.

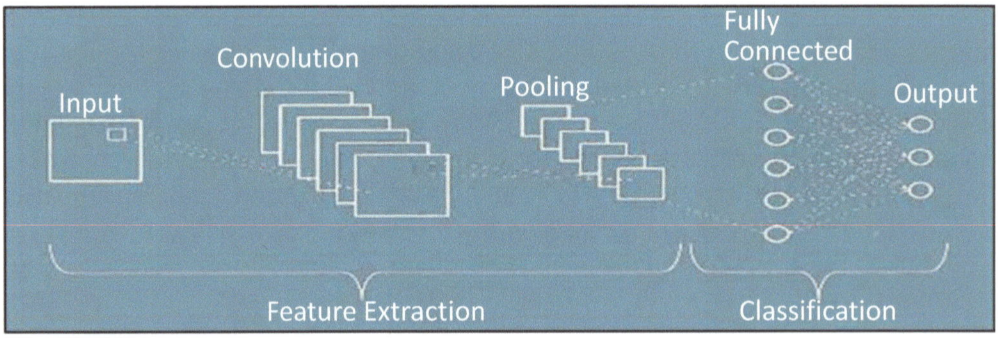

Fig. (9). Convolutional Neural Networks Architecture [45].

Use of Hidden State: All computations performed in a neural network are carried out at the hidden layer, where statistical parameters are utilized, along with an activation function. Mathematically, this can be represented as:

H(y) = activation (wi * x(y) + v * h(y-1) + b) (3)

Where H(y) represents the hidden state at time step y. X(y) represents the input at time step y, wi represents the weight matrix for the current input, v represents the weight matrix for the previous hidden state, and b represents the bias vector.

Activation represents an activation function like RELU.

- Output generation: The output layer is used to generate an output or prediction. This can be done using a fully connected layer connected with the hidden state, followed by an activation function if needed.
- Vanishing and exploding gradients: Conversely, exploding gradients can cause instability. Techniques like gradient clipping and specialized activation functions (like ISTM and GRU) are designed to mitigate these issues.
- Convergence and balance: The ideal state for GANN training is that it has the ability to classify both real and generated data with a 50% probability. However, achieving this balance can be challenging, and the training process can be sensitive to hyperparameters.
- Variations and advances: Since the introduction of GAN, several variations and improvements have been proposed, including conditional GANs, Wasserstein GANs (WGANs), CycleGANs, StyleGANs, and more. These variations address specific challenges and tasks, making GANS more versatile and practical.
- Autoencoders: Autoencoders are used in such neural networks where unsupervised learning is being used. These networks comprise encoder maps that map the inputs to the respective lower dimensions. They are also used for anomaly detection, noise reduction, and classification.
- Reinforcement learning networks: Reinforcement learning networks are used for making decisions according to the environment where the agent has been placed. Each architecture is tailored to specific tasks and data types, and researchers continually explore new variations and improvements to these classifiers.

KEY CHALLENGES

This section examines the multifaceted role of deep learning in healthcare and its impact on reshaping the medical practice landscape. At the forefront of deep learning's contributions to healthcare is its capacity to analyze medical images with unparalleled precision. Radiology and medical imaging, critical for diagnosing conditions ranging from cancer to neurological disorders, have greatly benefited from deep learning algorithms. These algorithms can detect subtle abnormalities that might evade human eyes, enabling earlier and more accurate diagnoses. Moreover, by continuously learning from new data, these models improve over time, ensuring consistently high diagnostic accuracy. Various challenges need to be addressed before applying deep neural network algorithms in the healthcare domain.

- Data security: It is crucial to understand that the personal information of every patient is sensitive and it must be secured with great care to avoid any harm. Many security breaches are reported nowadays.

- Data quality and bias: Healthcare data can be noisy, incomplete, and biased. The noise and the ability to make biased predictions and decisions potentially exacerbate healthcare disparities.
- Interoperability: Healthcare systems often use different data formats and standards. Integrating deep learning models into existing healthcare infrastructure can be challenging due to issues related to data interoperability and standardization.
- Scalability: Deep learning approaches used in large neural networks are often computationally intensive and may not scale easily. Deploying such models in real-time healthcare settings, such as hospitals, can be resource-intensive.
- Explainability and interpretability: In healthcare, where the stakes are high, it is crucial to explain model predictions to gain the trust of both patients and doctors.
- Regulatory approval: Deep learning models used in healthcare may require regulatory approval, a process that can be lengthy and costly.
- Healthcare validation: Validating deep learning models for clinical use is essential but can be complex and time-consuming. It involves demonstrating that the model's predictions improve patient outcomes and align with clinical guidelines.
- Data imbalance: In healthcare, certain conditions or outcomes may be rare, leading to imbalanced datasets.
- Continuous learning and adaptation: Healthcare is a dynamic field with evolving practices and guidelines. Robust strategies for data collection, preprocessing, model validation, and ethical considerations are essential to understand the potential of advanced technologies.

CONCLUSION

In summary, this chapter offers a comprehensive exploration of lung diseases, systematically categorizing them based on anatomical impact and reviewing pertinent literature to contextualize current understanding. It further elucidates the foundational principles of deep learning, detailing its algorithms, applications, and transformative role in modern healthcare. By examining how deep learning enhances disease detection and prevention, and by surveying existing research and implementation challenges, the chapter underscores both the promise and complexity of integrating artificial intelligence into clinical practice. Collectively, the insights presented herein serve as a valuable resource for researchers, practitioners, and policymakers seeking to advance data-driven approaches in pulmonary medicine and beyond.

REFERENCES

[1] Spagnolo P, Ryerson CJ, Guler S, *et al.* Occupational interstitial lung diseases. J Intern Med 2023; 294(6): 798-815.
[http://dx.doi.org/10.1111/joim.13707] [PMID: 37535448]

[2] National Toxicology Program. National Institute of Environmental Health Sciences. National Institutes of Health, U.S. Department of Health and Human Services, Research Triangle Park, NC. Chemical Information Review Document for Arbutin [CAS No. 497-76-7] and Extracts from Arctostaphylos uva-ursi: Supporting Nomination for Toxicological Evaluation by the National Toxicology Program. 2006 Jan.

[3] Cui Q, Carruthers S, McIvor A, Smaill F, Thabane L, Smieja M. Effect of smoking on lung function, respiratory symptoms and respiratory diseases amongst HIV-positive subjects: a cross-sectional study. AIDS Res Ther 2010; 7(1): 6.
[http://dx.doi.org/10.1186/1742-6405-7-6] [PMID: 20298614]

[4] Falcon-Rodriguez CI, Osornio-Vargas AR, Sada-Ovalle I, Segura-Medina P. Aeroparticles, composition, and lung diseases. Front Immunol 2016; 7: 3.
[http://dx.doi.org/10.3389/fimmu.2016.00003] [PMID: 26834745]

[5] Brenner DR, McLaughlin JR, Hung RJ. Previous lung diseases and lung cancer risk: A systematic review and meta-analysis. PLoS One 2011; 6(3): e17479.
[http://dx.doi.org/10.1371/journal.pone.0017479] [PMID: 21483846]

[6] Wardlaw TM, Johansson EW, Hodge MJ. Pneumonia: The forgotten killer of children. UNICEF; 2006.

[7] Wunderink RG, Waterer G. Advances in the causes and management of community acquired pneumonia in adults. BMJ 2017; 358: j2471.
[http://dx.doi.org/10.1136/bmj.j2471] [PMID: 28694251]

[8] Tobias RR, De Jesus LC, Mital ME, *et al.* RIVF International Conference on Computing and Communication Technologies (RIVF) 2020; 1-6.

[9] Stephen O, Sain M, Maduh UJ, Jeong DU. An efficient deep learning approach to pneumonia classification in healthcare. J Healthc Eng 2019; 2019(1): 1-7.
[http://dx.doi.org/10.1155/2019/4180949] [PMID: 31049186]

[10] Sasikaladevi N, Revathi A. Intelligent prognostic system for pediatric pneumonia based on sustainable IoHT. Multimedia Tools Appl 2023; 82(17): 26901-17.
[http://dx.doi.org/10.1007/s11042-023-14930-z]

[11] Chouhan V, Singh SK, Khamparia A, *et al.* A novel transfer learning based approach for pneumonia detection in chest X-ray images. Appl Sci (Basel) 2020; 10(2): 559.
[http://dx.doi.org/10.3390/app10020559]

[12] Kermany DS, Goldbaum M, Cai W, Valentim CC, Liang H, Baxter SL, McKeown A, Yang G, Wu X, Yan F, Dong J. Identifying medical diagnoses and treatable diseases by image-based deep learning cell. 2018 Feb 22;172(5):1122-31.

[13] Rahman T, Chowdhury MEH, Khandakar A, *et al.* Transfer learning with deep Convolutional Neural Network (CNN) for pneumonia detection using chest X-ray. Appl Sci (Basel) 2020; 10(9): 3233.
[http://dx.doi.org/10.3390/app10093233]

[14] Rajpurkar P. CheXNet: Radiologist-level pneumonia detection on chest x-rays with deep learning. ArXiv abs/1711. 2017;5225.

[15] Ayan E, Ünver HM. Diagnosis of pneumonia from chest X-ray images using deep learning. In 2019, a Scientific meeting on electrical-electronics & biomedical engineering and computer science (EBBT) 2019 Apr 24 (pp. 1-5). Ieee.

[16] Gupta A, Sheth P, Xie P. Neural architecture search for pneumonia diagnosis from chest X-rays. Sci

Rep [Internet]. 2022;12(1):11309. Available from: https://doi.org/10.1038/s41598-022-15341-0

[17] Kumar Acharya A, Satapathy R. A deep learning based approach towards the automatic diagnosis of pneumonia from chest radiographs. Biomed Pharmacol J 2020; 13(1): 449-55. [http://dx.doi.org/10.13005/bpj/1905]

[18] Elshennawy NM, Ibrahim DM. Deep-pneumonia framework using deep learning models based on chest X-ray images. Diagnostics (Basel) 2020; 10(9): 649. [http://dx.doi.org/10.3390/diagnostics10090649] [PMID: 32872384]

[19] Hurt B, Yen A, Kligerman S, Hsiao A. Augmenting interpretation of chest radiographs with deep learning probability maps. J Thorac Imaging 2020; 35(5): 285-93. [http://dx.doi.org/10.1097/RTI.0000000000000505] [PMID: 32205817]

[20] J. Young and A. Suryadibrata, "Applicability of various pre-trained deep convolutional neural networks for pneumonia classification based on x-ray images," Int. J. Adv. Trends Comput. Sci. Eng., pp. 2649–2654, 2020. [http://dx.doi.org/10.30534/ijatcse/2020/24932020]

[21] World Health Organization. Global status report on alcohol and health 2018. World Health Organization 2018.

[22] Arja A, Tadesse S, Agachew M, *et al.* The burden of tuberculosis across regions in Ethiopia: A systematic subnational analysis for the global burden of disease study 2019. Ethiop J Health Dev 2023; 37(2)

[23] Melendez J, van Ginneken B, Maduskar P, *et al.* A novel multiple-instance learning-based approach to computer-aided detection of tuberculosis on chest X-rays. IEEE Trans Med Imaging 2015; 34(1): 179-92. [http://dx.doi.org/10.1109/TMI.2014.2350539] [PMID: 25163057]

[24] Vajda S, Karargyris A, Jaeger S, *et al.* Feature selection for automatic tuberculosis screening in frontal chest radiographs. J Med Syst 2018; 42(8): 146. [http://dx.doi.org/10.1007/s10916-018-0991-9] [PMID: 29959539]

[25] Sandal A, Akgün M, de Bellevaux BN. Occupational Lung Diseases. Airway diseases. Cham: Springer International Publishing 2023; pp. 1-37. [http://dx.doi.org/10.1007/978-3-031-22483-6_96-1]

[26] Goobie GC, Li X, Ryerson CJ, Carlsten C, Johannson KA, Fabisiak JP, *et al.* PM2.5 and constituent component impacts on global DNA methylation in patients with idiopathic pulmonary fibrosis. Environ Pollut. 2023;318:120942. [http://dx.doi.org/10.1016/j.envpol.2022.120942] [PMID: 36574806]

[27] Cui Q. EFFECT OF SMOKING AND CESSATION IN HIV-INFECTED PEOPLE. In 2011. Available from: https://api.semanticscholar.org/CorpusID:70728540

[28] Losacco C, Perillo A. Particulate matter air pollution and respiratory impact on humans and animals. Environ Sci Pollut Res [Internet]. 2018;25(34): 33901-10. [http://dx.doi.org/10.1007/s11356-018-3344-9]

[29] Liang H-Y, Li X-L, Yu X-S, Guan P, Yin Z-H, He Q-C, et al. Facts and fiction of the relationship between preexisting tuberculosis and lung cancer risk: A systematic review. Int J Cancer [Internet]. 2009 Dec 15;125(12): 2936-44. Available from: https://doi.org/10.1002/ijc.24636

[30] Wardlaw TM, Johansson EW, Hodge MJ. Pneumonia: the forgotten killer of children. UNICEF, 2006.

[31] Cao B, Huang Y, She D-Y, Cheng Q-J, Fan H, Tian X-L, *et al.* Diagnosis and treatment of community-acquired pneumonia in adults: 2016 clinical practice guidelines by the Chinese Thoracic Society, Chinese Medical Association. Clin Respir J [Internet]. 2018 Apr 1;12(4): 1320-60. Available from: https://doi.org/10.1111/crj.12674

[32] Tobias RR, De Jesus LC, Mital ME, *et al.* RIVF International Conference on Computing and

Communication Technologies (RIVF) 2020; 1-6.

[33] Hashmi MF, Katiyar S, Keskar AG, Bokde ND, Geem ZW. Efficient pneumonia detection in chest xray images using deep transfer learning. Diagnostics. 2020;10(6): 1-23. [http://dx.doi.org/10.3390/diagnostics10060417]

[34] Ayan E, Ünver HM. Diagnosis of pneumonia from chest X-ray images using deep learning. In 2019, Scientific meeting on Electrical-Electronics & Biomedical Engineering and Computer Science (EBBT), 2019, Apr 24 (pp. 1-5). Ieee.

[35] Mann PS, Panchal SD, Singh S, Saggu GS, Gupta K. A hybrid deep convolutional neural network model for improved diagnosis of pneumonia. Neural Comput Appl [Internet]. 2024; 36(4): 1791-804. Available from: https://doi.org/10.1007/s00521-023-09147-y

[36] Kermany DS, Goldbaum M, Cai W, et al. Identifying medical diagnoses and treatable diseases by image-based deep learning. Cell 2018; 172(5): 1122-1131.e9. [http://dx.doi.org/10.1016/j.cell.2018.02.010] [PMID: 29474911]

[37] Ullah MS, Qayoom H, Hassan F. Viral Pneumonia Detection Using Modified GoogleNet Through Lung X-rays. In: 2021 4th International Symposium on Advanced Electrical and Communication Technologies (ISAECT). 2021. p. 1-6. [http://dx.doi.org/10.1109/ISAECT53699.2021.9668553]

[38] Rajpurkar P. CheXNet: Radiologist-Level Pneumonia Detection on Chest X-Rays with Deep Learning. ArXiv abs/1711. 2017;5225.

[39] Ayan E, Ünver HM. Diagnosis of pneumonia from chest X-ray images using deep learning. In 2019, Scientific meeting on electrical-electronics & biomedical engineering and computer science (EBBT) 2019 Apr 24 (pp. 1-5). Ieee.

[40] Ghuse ND, Monga S. A Review on Pneumonia Detection Using Artificial Intelligence Techniques. In: 2024 2nd International Conference on Artificial Intelligence and Machine Learning Applications Theme: Healthcare and Internet of Things (AIMLA). 2024. p. 1-5. [http://dx.doi.org/10.1109/AIMLA59606.2024.10531467]

[41] Maghdid HS, Asaad AT, Ghafoor KZ, Sadiq AS, Mirjalili S, Khan MK. Diagnosing COVID-19 pneumonia from x-ray and CT images using deep learning and transfer learning algorithms. In: ProcSPIE [Internet]. 2021. p. 117340E. Available from: https://doi.org/10.1117/12.2588672

[42] Tsai M-J, Tao Y-H. Deep learning technology Applied to medical image tissue classification. Diagnostics. 2022; 12(10): 2430. [http://dx.doi.org/10.3390/diagnostics12102430]

[43] Rajeashwari S, Arunesh K. Enhancing pneumonia diagnosis with ensemble-modified classifier and transfer learning in deep-CNN based classification of chest radiographs. Biomed Signal Process Control [Internet]. 2024; 93: 106130. Available from: https://www.sciencedirect.com/science/article/pii/S1746809424001885

[44] Salehi S, Abedi A, Radmard AR, Sorouri M, Gholamrezanezhad A. Chest computed tomography manifestation of coronavirus disease 2019 (COVID-19) in patients with cardiothoracic conditions. J Thorac Imaging 2020; 35(4): W90-6. [http://dx.doi.org/10.1097/RTI.0000000000000531] [PMID: 32404799]

[45] Young JC, Suryadibrata A. Applicability of various pre-trained deep convolutional neural networks for pneumonia classification based on x-ray images. Int J 2020; 9(3)

[46] Sotgiu G, Sulis G, Matteelli A. Tuberculosis—A world health organization perspective. Tuberculosis and Nontuberculous Mycobacterial Infections. 2017 Jun 1:211-28.

[47] World Health Organization. Global tuberculosis report 2021: supplementary material. World Health Organization; 2022 Mar 31.

[48] Heo SJ, Kim Y, Yun S, *et al.* Deep learning algorithms with demographic information help to detect

tuberculosis in chest radiographs in annual workers' health examination data. Int J Environ Res Public Health 2019; 16(2): 250.
[http://dx.doi.org/10.3390/ijerph16020250] [PMID: 30654560]

[49] Cao Y, Liu C, Liu B, *et al.* 2016.Improving tuberculosis diagnostics using deep learning and mobile health technologies among resource-poor and marginalized communities.
[http://dx.doi.org/10.1109/CHASE.2016.18]

[50] Becker AS, Blüthgen C, Phi van VD, *et al.* Detection of tuberculosis patterns in digital photographs of chest X-ray images using Deep Learning: feasibility study. Int J Tuberc Lung Dis 2018; 22(3): 328-35.
[http://dx.doi.org/10.5588/ijtld.17.0520] [PMID: 29471912]

[51] Hooda R, Mittal A, Sofat S. Automated TB classification using ensemble of deep architectures. Multimedia Tools Appl 2019; 78(22): 31515-32.
[http://dx.doi.org/10.1007/s11042-019-07984-5]

[52] Melendez J, Sánchez CI, Philipsen RHHM, *et al.* An automated tuberculosis screening strategy combining X-ray-based computer-aided detection and clinical information. Sci Rep 2016; 6(1): 25265.
[http://dx.doi.org/10.1038/srep25265] [PMID: 27126741]

[53] Petty TL. The history of COPD. Int J Chron Obstruct Pulmon Dis 2006; 1(1): 3-14.
[http://dx.doi.org/10.2147/copd.2006.1.1.3] [PMID: 18046898]

[54] Gluecker T, Capasso P, Schnyder P, *et al.* Clinical and radiologic features of pulmonary edema. Radiographics 1999; 19(6): 1507-31.
[http://dx.doi.org/10.1148/radiographics.19.6.g99no211507] [PMID: 10555672]

[55] Kim CFB, Jackson EL, Woolfenden AE, *et al.* Identification of bronchioalveolar stem cells in normal lung and lung cancer. Cell 2005; 121(6): 823-35.
[http://dx.doi.org/10.1016/j.cell.2005.03.032] [PMID: 15960971]

[56] Wells AU, Hirani N, Egan JJ, *et al.* Interstitial lung disease guideline. Thorax 2008; 63 (Suppl. 5): v1-v58.
[http://dx.doi.org/10.1136/thx.2008.101691] [PMID: 18757459]

CHAPTER 5

Wearable Healthcare

Neeraj Gupta[1,*]

[1] *Department of Information Technology, Panipat Institute of Engineering and Technology, Samalka, Haryana, India*

Abstract: The increasing global population, climate change, aging and chronic diseases, availability of healthcare facilities in selected cities and towns, and increasing cost of medical expenses are just a few reasons that are driving transitions from traditional hospital-based systems to individual-centric healthcare systems. With advancements in the semiconductor industry, material science, and data science, wearable technology has seen noticeable advancement and growth. The chapter aims to cover the technical aspects involved in wearable technology. The work delved deep into the architecture aspects, energy harvesting and management, and data processing cycle, forming the technological backbone for monitoring and transferring vital body signals to remote locations. The aggregate information helps detect, prevent, and monitor diseases in healthcare. The chapter thoroughly discusses the wearable type in healthcare and the latest devices commercially available for consumption in the healthcare industry. The chapter highlights thc limitations and challenges hindering their availability at the grassroots population level. This chapter aims to ensure that technological advancements can be comfortable and healthy for ordinary people.

Keywords: Computing, Human, Healthcare, Sensors, Wearable.

INTRODUCTION

The human race has made sustained efforts toward the longevity of human life. Present medical facilities do not come at an affordable cost to ordinary people, especially in third-world countries. Technology intervention is required to ensure affordable healthcare. ICT-based healthcare in post-COVID times has caught the attention of the government, scientific communities, and academia. A possible solution is using numerous IoT sensors that can communicate with each other and are backed by cloud services for the collection and analysis of data.

Wearable technologies are the next megatrend that aims to provide reasonably priced healthcare to patients [1]. Different authors have defined wearables based on their application area, and there is no standard way of defining wearable

* **Corresponding author Neeraj Gupta:** Department of Information Technology, Panipat Institute of Engineering and Technology, Samalka, Haryana, India; E-mail: neeraj.it@piet.co.in

Neeraj Gupta, Abdelhameed Ibrahim, Bhavesh Vyas & Shobhna Jeet (Eds.)

technology. The two most appropriate definitions, considering the vast applications of wearable are:

- "An application-enabled computing device that accepts and processes inputs. This device is a fashion accessory usually worn or attached to the body. The device could work independently or be tethered to a smartphone, allowing some meaningful interaction with the user. The wearable product could be on the body (like a smart patch), around the body (like a wristwatch or a headband), or in the body (like an identification sensor embedded under the skin or a sensor attached to the heart monitoring cardiac aberrations)" [2].
- "Small electronic and mobile devices, or computers with wireless communications capability that are incorporated into gadgets, accessories, or clothes, which can be worn on the human body, or even invasive versions such as micro-chips or smart tattoos" [3]

The report published on July 8, 2024 [4] reported that globally, the value of wearable technology was USD 120.54 billion, projected to be USD 1695.46 billion by 2032. Considering the usage of wearables across different segments, healthcare wearable devices globally account for 25% of the market share. The report [5] suggested that the healthcare wearable market would be USD 61.30 in 2022. For the forecast period 2023-2030, the report predicted the market will expand at a compound annual growth rate of 14.6%. These wearables can be broadly categorized into four classes:

- Carried
- Mounted
- Intimate
- Embedded

Smartphones are classified as carry wearables since they can be carried and are close to the body. Mounted devices like smartwatches, glasses, and mounted displays are worn, and they monitor vital parameters that can be collected through the organs. Devices almost indistinguishable from the human body, like prostheses and contact lenses, are termed intimate devices. Finally, wearables embedded inside the human body are examples of embedded technologies.

This chapter delves into various aspects of wearables in healthcare. Section 2 discusses wearable architecture. Section 3 highlights energy harvesting and its management. Section 4 delves into critical elements of the data processing cycle. Section 5 illustrates various applications in the healthcare industry. Section 6 discusses the limitations and challenges of wearable technology.

ARCHITECTURE

The wearable technology is woven around the Internet of Things (IoT) ecosystem. Body sensors, Body Area Networks, Fog Computing / Edge Computing, Mist Computing, and Cloud Computing are vital components of wearable IoT (WIoT). Two prominent IoT architectures that standardize communication between various devices are 1. The oneM2M architecture model [6] and 2. The IoT World Forum architecture. Both architectures intend to ease the interoperability among heterogeneous devices, services, and applications.

Wearable Body Sensors

Wearable Body Sensors (WBS) are miniature sensors capable of data collection, computing, communication, storage, and energy management. The primary requirements while deploying WBS are [7]:

- Accurate data is collected either directly through sensors or indirectly through peripheral devices. The health parameters being monitored are vital for medication during routine and emergency patient situations. Devices must meet global standards before they are deployed for data supervision and management.
- It is imperative to process the collected data locally or remotely for necessary feedback and to activate the response system. WBSs have very limited computing power and storage capacity. The vast amount of data generated must be stored and computed at the remote end. However, communication delays can cause devices to respond too slowly when a patient's vital signs become unstable.

Fig. (**1**) illustrates the applications and categorization of the wearable sensors.

Body Area Network

In the literature, Body Area Networks are IEEE 802.15.6 compliant networks, sometimes called Body Sensor Networks, Medical Body Area Networks, and Wireless Body Area Networks. BAN refers to very short-range communication by biosensors on, near, within, and around the body. The network is connected to an Internet Gateway, ensuring continuous real-time medical data aggregation and monitoring. The deployed sensors must perform their intended operations and update the patient's live location. The typical BAN consists of sensors, processors, transceivers, and batteries. The key challenges that need to be addressed are:

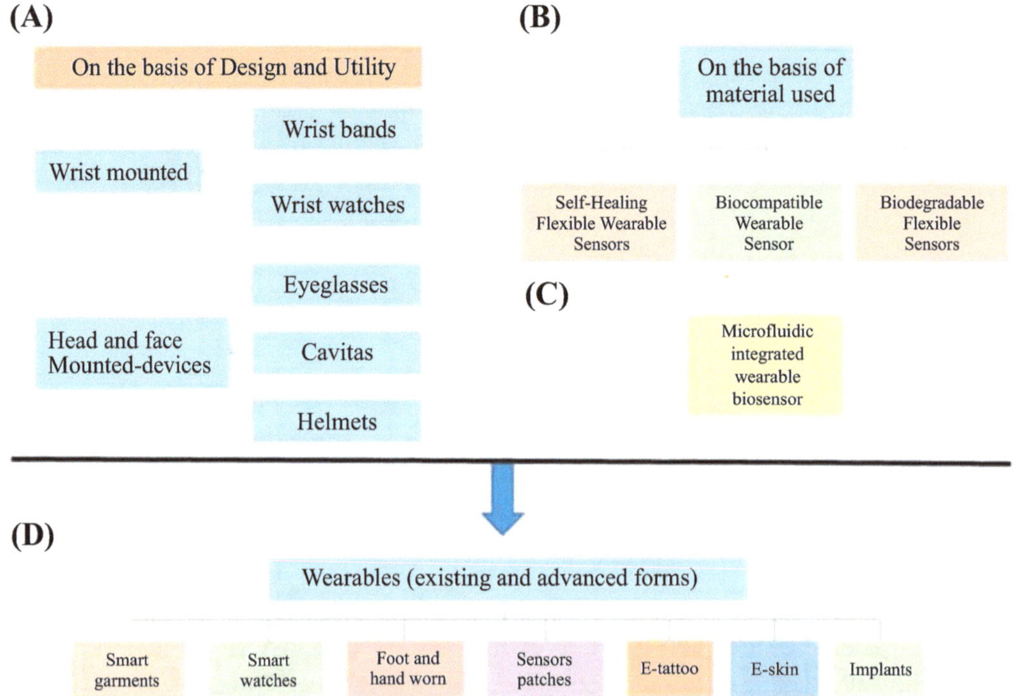

Fig. (1). Various categorization of wearables [8].

- Data Quality: Data quality needs to be high to facilitate the right and appropriate decision-making. Deployments must be thoroughly tested and validated before deployment. Consistent performance is a prime consideration for the WBAN.
- Data Management: Sensors generate a huge volume of data. Patient data management is a vital issue that needs to be addressed.
- Security: The patient data being communicated is personal, and any data breach directly affects the patient's privacy. Efforts should be directed to ensure interference and secure communication between various heterogeneous devices and networks. The devices in BAN are resource-constrained, so existing security solutions cannot be directly applied.
- Energy: The sensors dissipate energy during data collection and communication. The body sensors are energy-constrained, so saving the devices' power is essential. The accuracy of data during collection and communication is hugely dependent on the device's power. Energy management and utilization are crucial issues in wearable technology.

Cloud Computing

Wireless sensor networks are based on a client-server architecture. The sensor data was communicated to a central server for further processing. In case of wearables, the voluminous unstructured data is collected across different users for its dissemination. The most logical solution is to shift to the cloud. The prime advantages are:

- Depending upon the usage, the application could be served as a service.
- The computing and storage can be consolidated as a centralized entity.
- The ubiquitous nature of the cloud enables the healthcare worker to monitor the patient's parameters from any location.
- The multitenant facility in cloud storage ensures that users' privacy and security are maintained.

However, bandwidth, distance, and a complete lack of internet service could jeopardize the delay in activating the desired IoT unit or service during the needed hours. Smart wearables are emerging quickly, and requirements such as fast processing, more storage, conserving bandwidth, and increased efficiency must be met.

Fog Computing

It is preferable to have a decentralized computing architecture that could accommodate the requirements of the IoT ecosystem, especially wearable technology. Fog computing provides computing, storage, and networking services between the end devices and cloud data centers. Routers, IoT gateways, integrated access devices, multiplexers, and similar edge devices are key elements for providing services to edge devices. Since the generated data is unstructured, the idea is to process the data by the units collocated near the generating sensors. The semi-processed data can be forwarded to the cloud data centers, reducing the latency and processing requirements. Fog devices, being closer to multiple heterogeneous devices, can support data contextualization more. This becomes critical in identifying the patterns that may be otherwise omitted, thus supporting a more informed decision process at the local level.

Mist Computing

Edge computing can be divided into Fog Computing and Mist Computing [9] as shown in Fig. (**2**). The idea is to push decision-making to the lowest part of the hierarchy: the devices and IoT devices. With state-of-the-art technology in microprocessors, microcontrollers, and sensor technology, the devices can perform low-level data filtering and analytical computations.

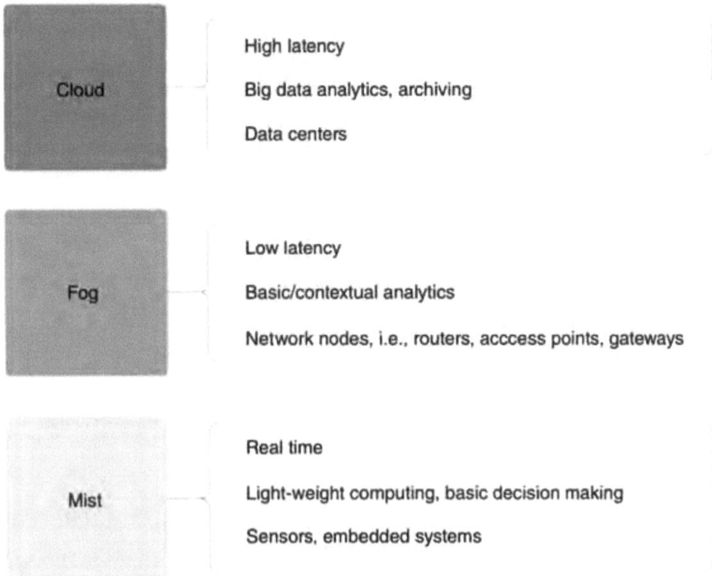

Fig. (2). Broad use case of cloud, fog, and mist computing [9].

Fog and Mist computing are complementary technologies that support cloud computing. Time-sensitive applications can be better supported at the local layer of the architectural framework. Bi-filtered data can be aggregated as historical data for big data analysis and long-term storage.

As illustrated in Fig. (**3**), the four-layer architecture is the appropriate architecture considering the present IoT ecosystem. The bottom-most layer is the user. The second layer will comprise users' wearable sensors that are responsible for collecting the data. The generated data will be communicated to the IoT gateway. The gateway is either embedded into the sensors (like smartphones) or could be connected through wireless communication (like Bluetooth). These gateways include an application that can perform low-level analytics, visualization, and user interaction. The fog devices forward the data to the cloud data centers for further processing. The processed data can be sent as feedback to users so they can make decisions.

ENERGY HARVESTING AND MANAGEMENT

Wearables are dependent on power sources to ensure their longevity. It is important to delve into issues concerning energy harvesting, energy storage, and optimal management to ensure that devices continue to work at their optimal level. Power-starved devices will generate unreliable data.

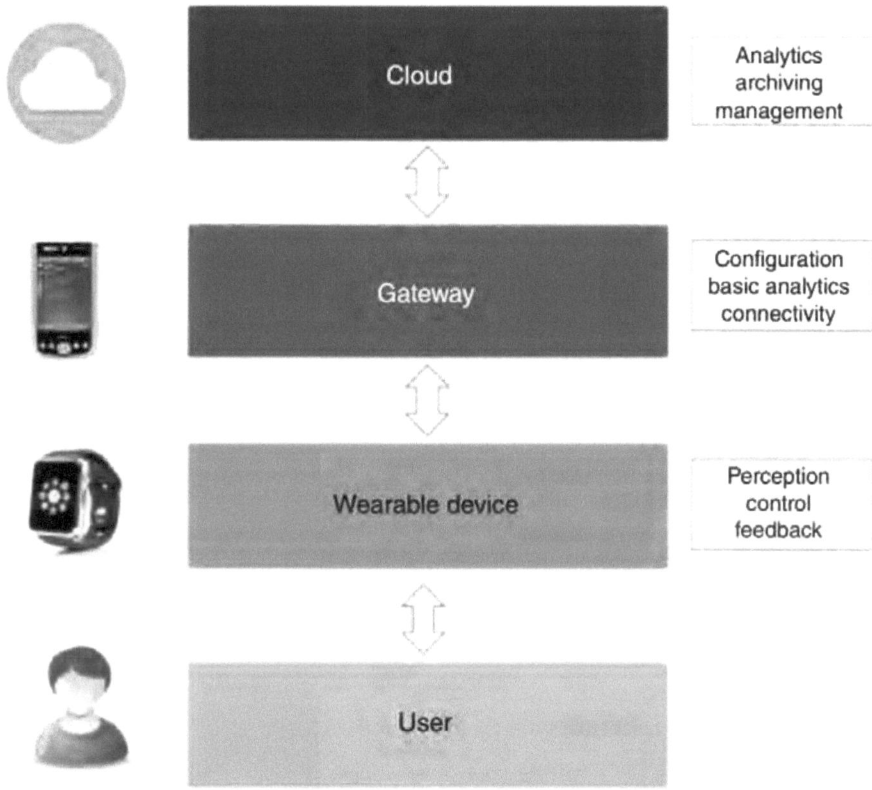

Fig. (3). Wearable architecture [9].

Energy Harvesting

Energy harvesting for wearables liberates the tiny sensors from their dependency on batteries. Some groundbreaking innovation in the field of material science allows wearables to generate their own power. The devices can convert the human body's movement and heat energy into power themselves [10, 11].

- Triboelectric Generators: Polydimethylsiloxane, a silicon material, generates an electric charge when subjected to mechanical stress like bending and stretching. The device generates enough power to operate.
- Piezoelectric Materials: These materials convert mechanical energy into electrical energy. They are commonly used in sensors and actuators. Researchers at UK Southampton, have developed a textile made from piezoelectric material to generate electric power from the movement of the human body.
- Human Sweat: Wei Gao at the California Institute of Technology developed a wearable human skin to measure parameters like heart rate, blood sugar, *etc*. The device absorbs human sweat and mixes it with atmospheric oxygen. The process

generates 1.5 to 3.8 volts to recharge the fuel cells and support data transmission.

- Solar Cells: The wearables are 3D-printed sensor arrays, hydrogel-coated electrodes, and micro-capacitors. They are powered and recharged by solar energy.
- Radio-frequency: "Rectenna" is a wearable device that can harvest energy from RF signals from Wi-Fi routers and/or cell towers. These devices consist of an antenna and rectifier circuits that convert RF signals into an electric current.

Ongoing research into waste energy harvesting is expected to drive the creation of efficient and sustainable wearables. Energy harvesting ensures freedom from batteries, reducing dependencies on non-renewables and making wearables more affordable in the long run.

Energy Management

Energy storage and management are crucial issues for wearable devices. The storage area and its management are highly dependent on the design and utility of the devices. For example, smartphones and smartwatches need to be powered by an external battery. These batteries need to be recharged to maintain the devices' optimal functioning. Depending on energy density, lifetime, and size, the designer can choose between Li-ion batteries or supercapacitors.

Similarly, there has been a variety of charging hardware and supporting software to manage the working of batteries. Materials like gallium-based liquids with high conductivity and biocompatibility can be used with liquid-metal polymers to develop a cyborg device that conforms to human body contours. The unique properties of 2D materials drive electronic applications that can be integrated with wearable devices. Except for critical elderly conditions and patients admitted to hospitals, there is little usage in monitoring the user's health parameters continuously. The devices should be sensitive to awakening from active sleep mode in case there are significant changes in the vital parameters of the users. The energy can be harvested and stored during the sleep period.

Photovoltaic harvesting is suitable for high-power consumption devices. Thermoelectric generates low energy, making it ideal for ultra-low power consumption wearables like smartwatches. Piezoelectric wearables are usually embedded in fibers used in textiles. Their use is appropriate where the conditions are hot and less humid. A hybridization of Thermoelectric and Photovoltaic technology is preferred for harvesting purposes. Energy storage choices heavily depend on the wearable devices' material and purpose. For example, noninvasive wearables like skin-based ones cannot use Li-ion batteries. For healthcare wearables, there is a need for wireless, battery-free implant sensors. It is recommended that maximum power point tracking circuits, along with impedance trackers, be used to facilitate energy management during harvesting and operation usage.

DATA PROCESSING CYCLE

An automated healthcare system using wearables generates voluminous data characterized by velocity, variety, variability, and veracity. The data needs to be processed to gain meaningful insights so that practitioners can make informed decisions. The data processing cycle is depicted in Fig. (**4**).

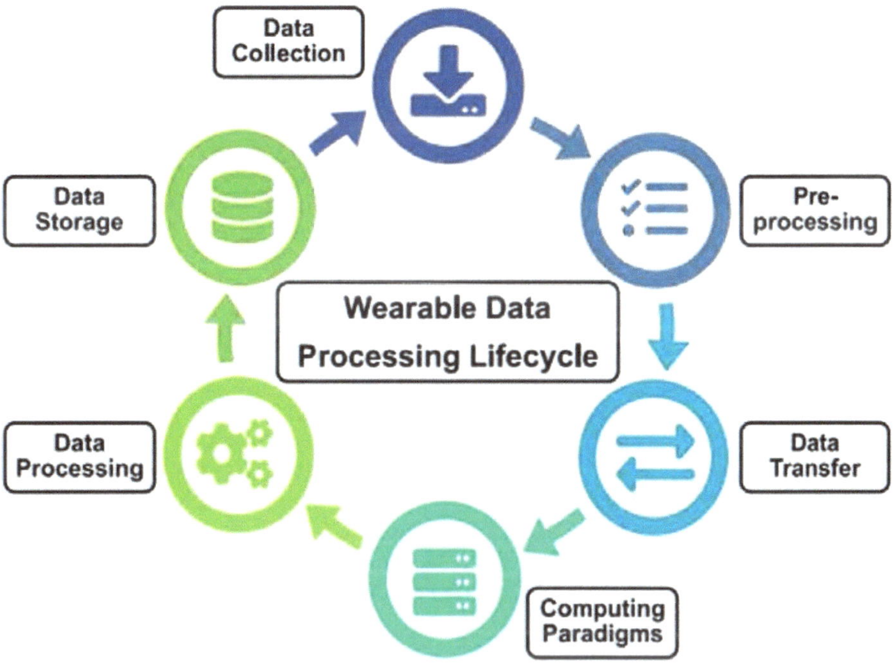
Data Collection
Pre-processing
Data Transfer
Computing Paradigms
Data Processing
Data Storage
Wearable Data Processing Lifecycle

Fig. (4). Wearable data processing life cycle [12].

Data Collection

The data collection process can be facilitated through crowd sensing [13]. Ubiquitous computing facilitates data collection through healthcare sensors monitoring millions of users globally. The collective data can be processed to extract information, analyze, and predict future actions. Crowd sensing can be broadly categorized as participatory crowdsensing [13] and opportunistic crowdsensing [14]. An individual actively shares the data with a community in participatory crowd sensing, such as sharing of COVID data through the mobile app. Opportunistic crowd sensing is more automated with no or minimal user actions. The wearable sensors can create autonomously opportunistic sensing networks to share data, location, and other essential information.

Preprocessing

Most of the data collected through wearable sensors is unstructured. Device performance can be affected by environmental issues, non-standardization, government regulation, transmission impairments, and other similar problems. The collected data can be plagued with duplicates, missing values, inconsistencies, errors, *etc*. It is essential to deal with data integration processes, specifically extraction and transformation before the data is stored in a data warehouse, cloud, or data lake.

The data needs to be preprocessed at each layer. The primary job should be able to standardize and transform into a representation that could be easily handled and stored. Data preprocessing is the most crucial step in the preparation process to avoid unnecessary computations and waste of storage. It is essential to clean and validate data from duplicates, outliers, missing values, and incomplete information. The preprocessing aims to improve data quality to ensure the machine can be reliably trained and the output validated. The 'informed' information displayed/shared with the users depends on the data quality to be analyzed.

Data Transfer

It is essential that data is communicated faithfully and securely to the desired endpoint. Data communication substantially drains the wearables' energy source, limiting the transmission encryption algorithm. The drained power source can also cause either loss of transmission or error-prone transmission. Readers are suggested to refer to section 3.4 of [12].

Computing Paradigms

The key architecture components have already been presented in Section 2. According to a study [15], the real computing architecture can be further classified as Mist Computing, Mobile Computing, Mobile Cloud Computing, Multi-access Edge Computing, and Mobile Ad Hoc Cloud Computing. Mobile computing refers to wireless mobile devices like smartphones, tablets, or similar devices running, as well as context-sensitive applications that can generate and communicate multimedia data, including audio and video. Mobile Ad Hoc cloud computing refers to a temporary network, like Bluetooth, created among several devices in communication range with each other. Multi-access edge computing is a network architecture that combines mobility, cloud services, and edge computing by making applications run in a decentralized fashion rather than from centralized cloud data centers. The main advantages are low latency, efficient networks, and a seamless user experience. Cloudlets are small cluster data centers available on the edge of the network to perform computation and speed up the performance of applications. They provide the platform infrastructure in terms of memory and processing power. The resources are delivered in the form of intelligent containers that are shared among the applications to maintain optimum desired performance.

Data Processing

Most of the wearable data can be classified under time-series [16]. The analysis of time-series data enables us to understand the past behavior of the series and helps in future predictions. Once sorted on the basis of time, the data can fluctuate due to the various components of the time series. Isolating multiple data components and their corresponding effect on the final analysis result is essential. The time series is helpful for classification, forecasting, and outlier detection. The collection of medical data is a time-consuming and tedious task. Data augmentation can aid in generating new data points using the previously available data. It is important to note that collected data may suffer from class imbalance and multivariate time series. Special augmentation techniques are needed to handle such data.

The recent advances in Deep Learning techniques have paved the way for more accurate analysis and predictions. Convolutional Neural Networks, Long Short-term Memory and its variants, Generative Adversarial Networks, Autoencoders, Reinforcement Learning, and Transfer Learning have been successfully applied and deployed to produce precise results. Libraries like XGBOOST, h2o, LightGBM, and CATBOOST have fastened data processing and helped achieve the desired outputs.

Data Storage

Data repositories store the processed data and feed the same to the recommendation systems for prediction and feedback purposes. Data is stored in data repositories. Data warehouses, data lakes, data marts, and cubes are key data management, storage, and reporting technologies.

APPLICATIONS IN THE HEALTHCARE INDUSTRY

The human body is complex, with intricate systems and processes working in tandem to maintain life and health. The human body parts generate many signals captured by physicians from ancient times to monitor vital signs of health. With the advent of modern science, various scientific devices are used to capture these key signals to determine the current state of human health. Fig. (**5**) depicts the inputs taken by the human body, the output generated by the human body, and the medical techniques used to monitor the generated signals by various body parts.

Fig. (**6**) illustrates various wearables developed for specific body parts to capture vital signals. This section covers the significant wearables that are commercially available for health monitoring purposes.

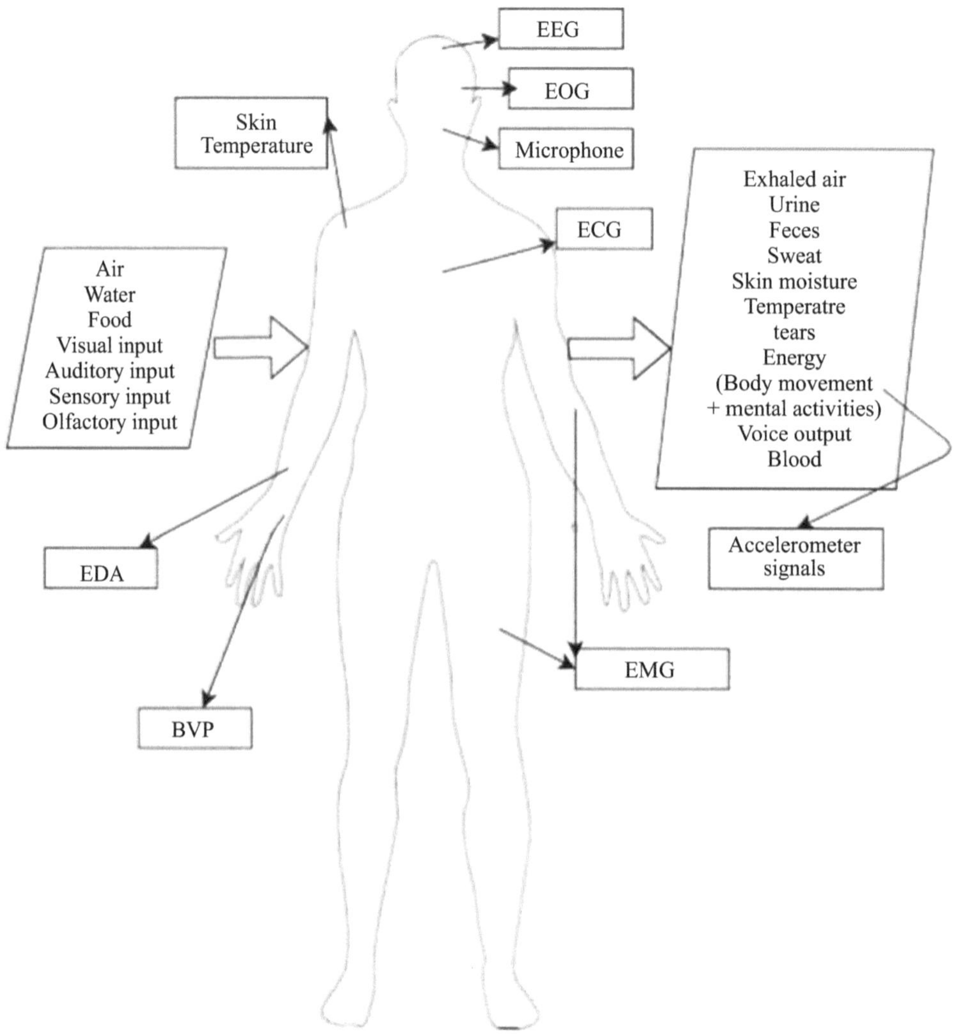

Fig. (5). Human body as systems and signal sources generated by various body parts [17].

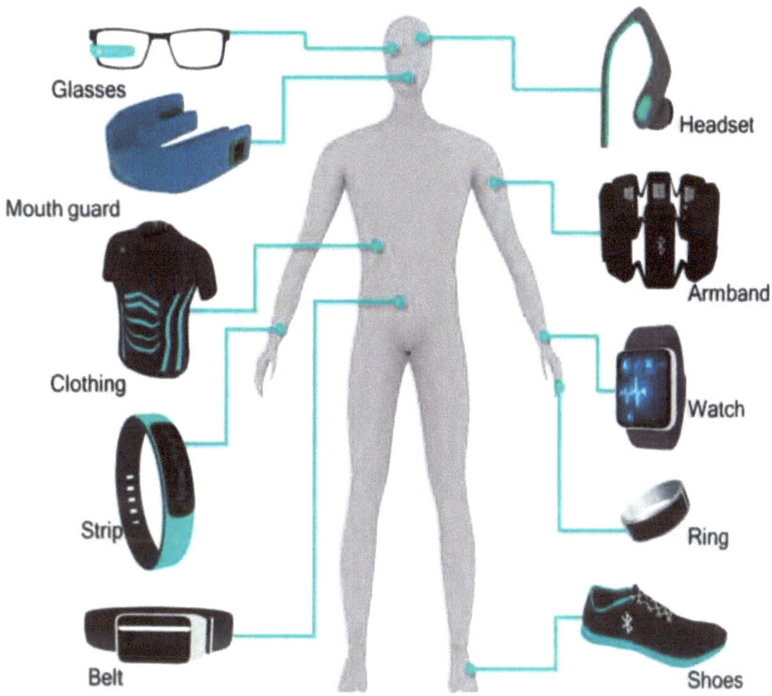

Fig. (6). Human wearable devices [18].

- Smart Thermometer: Thermometers can be classified based on how body temperature is measured: contact or contactless. Contact thermometers are based on integrated circuits and thermistors, while contactless thermometers are based on thermopiles and/or pyroelectric sensors [19]. These wearable thermometers are available in different sizes, costs, and forms. Wearable thermometers are being developed for other uses, including measuring skin temperature for detecting influenza, measuring menstrual cycle tracking, tracking heart rates, and many more. KINSA, Fitbit device, Oura Ring, and Whoop 4.0 are commercially available thermometers.
- Wristband: The wristbands are wearables that are worn on the wrist. The digital wristbands are capable of measuring pulse rate, body temperature, pulse rate, and blood pressure. Researchers used E4 wristbands developed by Empatica to detect and predict H1N1 influenza and the common cold (human rhinovirus) before its onset. The sensors could accurately measure body temperature, daily life activities, pulse rate, and body movement. Early detection ensures necessary intervention to stop the spread of viral respiratory infection in the community [20]. The Embrace Plus has replaced the E4. The new wearable can draw continuous data from EDA, PPG, accelerometer, and skin sensors. This device was co-designed by Emphatica, NASA, and HHS.

- Smart Watches: The smartwatches were not available for healthcare till 2012. Suunto M4 is the earliest smartwatch to monitor heart care and track physical activity. The Pebble smartwatch was the first breakthrough that paved the way for advanced health monitoring features [21]. Some of the best smartwatches that are available in the market are:
  - Apple Watch Series 9 is known for its comprehensive health tracking, including heart rate monitoring, ECG, blood oxygen levels, and menstrual cycle tracking.
  - Fitbit Sense 2 excels in stress management and sleep monitoring thanks to its advanced sensors and reliable sleep-tracking capabilities[1].
  - Samsung Galaxy Watch 7 offers body composition analysis, blood pressure monitoring, and a sleek design.
  - Withings ScanWatch features a premium design, an easy-to-use ECG monitor, and a long-lasting battery.
  - Garmin Venu 3 is known for its accurate GPS and heart rate sensors, sleep coaching, and on-device phone call support [22].

- Smart Glasses: Smart glasses or smart glasses are eye and head-worn wearable devices. Many smart glasses include displays that add information alongside what the wearer sees. Augmented reality-enabled smart glasses merge virtual information alongside the available physical information. The Head-mounted displays are predicted to reach US$5.1 billion in the health sector in the next decade [23]. Google Glass and Microsoft HoloLens are the two most prominent commercial gadgets available in the market. Google Glass combines eyeglasses with a high-definition camera to assist user interaction through voice commands. Microsoft HoloLens is based on AR technology that uses multiple sensors and holograms to create a simulated virtual world. The key medical applications of smart glasses are [24]:
  - Assisting medical education by virtualization of online information without interruption.
  - Assisting surgeries that are confined to small spaces and delicate anatomical structures.
  - Usefulness has been reported in the areas of autopsies, medical examination, and pathology.
  - The AR-assisted technology helps 3D projections find their application in telepathology and real-time pathology-radiology correlation.
  - Automatic recording of physical files in electronic medical record-compliant formats.
  - Smart contact lenses monitor various eye-related physiological functions. The first smart contact lens, the Tigger lens, was launched in 2016 to monitor glaucoma patients.
  - Smart Stethoscope: A stethoscope is one of the valuable tools for healthcare

professionals to assess and diagnose patients. It is an acoustic medical device for auscultation or listening to the internal sounds of the human body. With funding from NASA and the Bill & Melinda Gates Foundation, researchers, engineers, and doctors at Johns Hopkins University designed a smart Stethoscope [25]. The device uses digital sensing technology for sound capture, smart acoustics for noise cancellation, and AI to help healthcare patients make more accurate diagnoses. The work [26] devised a cost-effective intelligent stethoscope for cardiac auscultation. The device can record and send the signal to healthcare professionals remotely. AiSteth [27] is a commercially available stethoscope to screen, detect, and predict heart and lung diseases.

- Smart Patches: Smart patches are compact and noninvasive devices used to diagnose and monitor patients' vital signs. Smart patches are attached to the body with a skin adhesive that contains numerous sensors. They measure pulse rate, respiration rate, body temperature, and countless other parameters. The researchers have also developed a wearable skin patch that can measure the amount of insensible perspiration during the rest period [28]. This novel wearable applies to sports management, stress and tension monitoring, heat strokes, and other areas. In a groundbreaking advancement, Sheng Xu and the team at the University of California, San Diego, have developed a wearable ultrasound patch that enables continuous, noninvasive monitoring of blood flow in the brain. This innovative patch, which is soft and stretchy, can be comfortably worn on the temple and provides three-dimensional data on cerebral blood flow. The continuous monitoring capability of the patch addresses a critical gap in current clinical practices, offering a hands-free, consistent, and comfortable solution [29].
- A team of engineers has invented a soft, thin, stretchy device measuring just over 1 sq inch that can be attached to the skin outside the throat to help people with dysfunctional vocal cords regain their voice function [30].

Wearable technology has successfully addressed Smart Mood Monitoring Systems, Smart Rehabilitation systems, Smart Nutrition systems, and similar applications. COVID-19 has accelerated the pace of innovation in this sector. Wearables have been able to provide enhanced usability and seamless user experience compared to other classical portable devices.

LIMITATIONS AND CHALLENGES

Wearables for healthcare vary in size, shape, cost, features, accuracy, user experience, and technology. Some imperative questions enlist limitations and challenges that need to be addressed.

- Environmental Conditions: Environmental conditions vary widely worldwide. It is important that wearables are tested under varied conditions and samples. The final device should be tested for performance, function, and durability.
- User Experience: The user should be at ease while using these devices. The user's age is one considerable factor that determines the ease of usage. The necessary instructions should be given to the patient in the event of device failure, missing data, syncing the devices, or other technical problems. Sensors should be simple and easy to use.
- Specifications: The device should be compact, lightweight, optimized, and reliable. The device material should be biocompatible with the human body, especially for skin-based wearables. Implanted devices should be hermetically sealed to prevent the loss of liquids and chemicals. Any wearable should not obstruct the natural function and behaviors of the body parts. Depending on the user's lifestyle, any hazard associated with the device should be specifically stated.
- Metric: During the development phase, it is important to consider the metrics required for analysis and prediction purposes. Fig. (**1**) lists the categorization of wearable devices. Depending upon the wearable, the number of parameters will also vary. Output of the wearables must be duly validated against the medical gold standards. The regulating agencies should approve all commercials for local use. The sampling rate determines the available data samples for a machine learning algorithm to predict the outcome. The manufacturers should provide statistics, including sampling rate, algorithms deployed, number of parameters on which the machine is trained, and similar information in the public domain.
- Security: The data is communicated by wearable devices using short-range communication protocols like Zigbee, Bluetooth, RFID, and NFC. These protocols are not inherently secure. Security needs to be built at the upper layers to ensure that the confidentiality and privacy of the user data are maintained. Health and personal information collected are enormous amounts of data and are usually stored in the cloud. The critical question is to whom this data belongs: the user, the wearable company, the researchers, or the hospitals. It is equally important to enforce strong security features and legal frameworks to ensure that the integrity of data is always maintained.

- Standardization: Many wearable manufacturers enforce their own technology and protocols. A global standardization policy is needed to ensure compatibility among these devices.

CONCLUSION

The chapter presents a detailed analysis of the current state of affairs in the area of wearable technology. Wearables are a good combination of material science, electronics, and IoT to facilitate the monitoring of users' vital signs, provide first-hand information, and sometimes suggest medical advice in case of emergency. The pandemic has accelerated research in this area, though there is still a long way to go.

The area of cloud computing has matured, but from the wearables' point of view, edge computing and mist computing are the technologies to be focused upon. The federated learning should also be explored as it provides immense opportunities to share information and make more informed decisions. Energy is a prime requirement for any device to work correctly. In recent years, advancements in material science have been reported to help management in a noninvasive manner. There is a lot of research potential in this area that could be exploited.

The data processing cycle is well established and can be complemented by evolving technologies in the near future. Researchers have reported many wearables in the literature globally, but commercializing these devices is a big issue, especially in third-world countries. It has been reported [31] that Europe leads in research and innovations in wearable devices, but needs to provide a market for these devices. America provides a massive market for commercialized devices, but more research is required. Asia is reported to have stable growth in terms of research and usage. The study needs to report the data from the African and South American continents. Pricing will always be the most significant issue and roadblock to mass availability. The tremendous potential of wearables exists in villages and remote locations with insignificant medical facilities.

The work discusses and compares the most trending devices that have been reported and commercialized. Smartwatches are leading the sales of wearables in the present day. We have enlisted and elaborated on the limitations and challenges associated with wearables. Even in advanced countries, medical infrastructure was under immense pressure during pandemic times. There is immense potential to accelerate research and innovation to ensure affordable, accurate, precise, and improved health services reach remote parts of the world. IoMT technology can play a huge role in alleviating and bridging the challenges and enhancing more intelligent medical decision-making in the health sector.

REFERENCES

[1] Megatrends T. Technology Megatrends. 2024.

[2] Kurwa, M., Mohammed, A., & Liu W. Wearable technology, fashioning the future. [Internet]. 2008. Available from: http://www.flextronics.com/%0ADocuments/White papers/WT Fashioning the Future -%0AFINAL_AE.PDF

[3] Luczak T, Burch R, Lewis E, Chander H, Ball J. State-of-the-art review of athletic wearable technology: What 113 strength and conditioning coaches and athletic trainers from the USA said about

technology in sports. Int J Sport Sci \& Coach [Internet]. 2020;15(1):26–40. [http://dx.doi.org/10.1177/1747954119885244]

[4] Report H& SISMR. Wearable technology market size, share & industry analysis, by type (smart glasses, VR headsets, smart jackets and smart rings, smart watches, fit bands), by technology (IoT based, AR and VR, others), by end use (health and fitness, BFSI, gaming and enterainment, fashion, travel, education, and logistics & warehouse), and regional forecast, 2025-2023 [Internet]. 2024. Available from: https://www.fortunebusinessinsights.com/wearable-technology-market-106000

[5] 978-1-68038-165-8 RI. Wearable technology market size, share & trends analysis report by product (head & eyewear, wristwear), by application (consumer electronics, healthcare), by region (asia pacific, Europe), and segment forecasts, 2023 - 2030 [Internet]. 2023. Available from: https://www.grandviewresearch.com/industry-analysis/wearable-technology-market

[6] Using oneM2M [Internet]. [cited 2022 May 5]. Available from: https://onem2m.org/using-onem2m/developers/basics?jjj=1647576221153

[7] Hiremath S, Yang G, Mankodiya K. Wearable Internet of Things: Concept, Architectural Components and Promises for Person-Centered Healthcare. 2014; (August 2016).

[8] Sharma A, Badea M, Tiwari S, Marty JL. Wearable biosensors: An alternative and practical approach in healthcare and disease monitoring. Molecules 2021; 26(3): 748. [http://dx.doi.org/10.3390/molecules26030748] [PMID: 33535493]

[9] Architectures RH. Fundamentals of IoT and Wearable Technology Design. 2020; pp. 53-76. [http://dx.doi.org/10.1002/9781119617570.ch3]

[10] What are energy-harvesting wearables - Medical Buyer [Internet]. Medical Buyer. 2023 [cited 2024 Aug 4]. Available from: https://www.medicalbuyer.co.in/what-are-energy-harvesting-wearables/

[11] Julianne Pepitone. Energy Harvesting for Wearable Technology Steps Up Tiny worn devices won't need batteries thanks to these innovations. IEEE Spectrum [Internet]. 2023 Nov; Available from: https://spectrum.ieee.org/energy-harvesting-wearable-tech

[12] Ometov A, Shubina V, Klus L, *et al.* A Survey on Wearable Technology: History, State-of-the-Art and Current Challenges. Comput Netw 2021; 193(April): 108074. [http://dx.doi.org/10.1016/j.comnet.2021.108074]

[13] Raghu K. Ganti, Fan Ye and HL. Mobile Crowdsensing: Current State and Future Challenges. IEEE Commun Mag 2011; 32-9.

[14] Guo B, Wang Z, Yu Z, *et al.* Mobile Crowd Sensing and Computing. ACM Comput Surv 2015; 48(1): 1-31. [http://dx.doi.org/10.1145/2794400]

[15] Rius O. Cloud, Fog, and Edge Computing - Is this everything? [Internet]. 2020 [cited 2024 Aug 9]. Available from: https://www.e-zigurat.com/en/blog/beyond-cloud-fog-edge-computing/#comments

[16] Terzi M, Cenedese A, Susto GA. A multivariate symbolic approach to activity recognition for wearable applications. IFAC-PapersOnLine 2017; 50(1): 15865-70. [http://dx.doi.org/10.1016/j.ifacol.2017.08.2333]

[17] Sabry F, Eltaras T, Labda W, Alzoubi K, Malluhi Q. Machine Learning for Healthcare Wearable Devices: The Big Picture. J Healthc Eng. 2022;2022.

[18] Guk K, Han G, Lim J, *et al.* Evolution of wearable devices with real-time disease monitoring for personalized healthcare. Nanomaterials (Basel) 2019; 9(6): 813. [http://dx.doi.org/10.3390/nano9060813] [PMID: 31146479]

[19] Tamura T, Huang M, Togawa T. Current developments in wearable thermometers. Advanced Biomedical Engineering 2018; 7(0): 88-99. [http://dx.doi.org/10.14326/abe.7.88]

[20] Grzesiak E, Bent B, McClain MT, *et al.* Assessment of the feasibility of using noninvasive wearable

biometric monitoring sensors to detect influenza and the common cold before symptom onset. JAMA Netw Open 2021; 4(9): e2128534.
[http://dx.doi.org/10.1001/jamanetworkopen.2021.28534] [PMID: 34586364]

[21] Medical smartwatch: Wearable tech in healthcare [Internet]. 2023 [cited 2024 Aug 16]. Available from: https://www.arrow.com/en/research-and-events/articles/medical-smartwatch-technology-in-healthcare

[22] Walker A. The best smartwatches for keeping track of your health [Internet]. 2024. [cited 2024 Aug 16]. Available from: https://www.androidauthority.com/best-smartwatch-health-monitoring-3224222/

[23] Rahman R, Wood ME, Qian L, Price CL, Johnson AA, Osgood GM. Head-Mounted Display Use in Surgery: A Systematic Review. Surg Innov 2020; 27(1): 88-100.
[http://dx.doi.org/10.1177/1553350619871787] [PMID: 31514682]

[24] Baashar Y, Alkawsi G, Wan Ahmad WN, Alomari MA, Alhussian H, Tiong SK. Towards Wearable Augmented Reality in Healthcare: A Comparative Survey and Analysis of Head-Mounted Displays. Int J Environ Res Public Health 2023; 20(5): 3940.
[http://dx.doi.org/10.3390/ijerph20053940] [PMID: 36900951]

[25] HILALIEL M, West JE. A Smart Stethoscope Puts AI in Medics' Ears. IEEE Spectrum [Internet]. 2019; Available from: https://spectrum.ieee.org/a-smart-stethoscope-puts-ai-in-medics-ears

[26] Rao YS, Mehta B, Kathiriya A, Dharvia A, Pancholi D, Patel H. Smart Stethoscope for Remote Healthcare Monitoring Using IoT: A Cost-Effective Solution. In: 2023 3rd Asian Conference on Innovation in Technology (ASIANCON). 2023. p. 1–5.
[http://dx.doi.org/10.1109/ASIANCON58793.2023.10270283]

[27] AISTETH - SMART STETHOSCOPE [Internet]. Available from: https://aisteth.com/

[28] Ding H, Yang H, Tsujimura S. Nature-Inspired Superhydrophilic Biosponge as Structural Beneficial Platform for Sweating Analysis Patch. Adv Sci (Weinh) 2024; 11(30): 2401947. Available from: https://onlinelibrary.wiley.com/doi/abs/10.1002/advs.202401947
[http://dx.doi.org/10.1002/advs.202401947] [PMID: 38868908]

[29] Zhou S, Gao X, Park G, *et al.* Transcranial volumetric imaging using a conformal ultrasound patch. Nature 2024; 629(8013): 810-8.
[http://dx.doi.org/10.1038/s41586-024-07381-5] [PMID: 38778234]

[30] Lee CW. Speaking without vocal cords, thanks to a new AI-assisted wearable device [Internet]. 2024. Available from: https://newsroom.ucla.edu/releases/speaking-without-vocal-cords-ucla-engineering-wearable-tech

[31] Escobar-Linero E, Muñoz-Saavedra L, Luna-Perejón F, Sevillano JL, Domínguez-Morales M. Wearable Health Devices for Diagnosis Support: Evolution and Future Tendencies. Sensors (Basel) 2023; 23(3): 1678.
[http://dx.doi.org/10.3390/s23031678] [PMID: 36772718]

CHAPTER 6

Predicting the Risk of Heart Attack Using Machine Learning Algorithms

Maryam Shaaban[1] and **Abdelhameed Ibrahim**[1,*]

[1] *Faculty of Engineering, Design and Information & Communications Technology (EDICT), School of ICT, Bahrain Polytechnic, PO Box 33349, Isa Town, Bahrain*

Abstract: This chapter uses two datasets to predict heart attacks, which provide valuable insights into the machine learning algorithms used in the prediction process. The first dataset used in this chapter is the heart attack risk prediction dataset, which has 14 attributes relevant to heart health, including demographic information of the patient, clinical features, diagnostic test results, symptoms, risk factors, and outcome variables. The second dataset used in this chapter is the heart attack dataset collected at Zheen Hospital in Erbil, Iraq, in 2019. The dataset has 1319 records of patients and nine attributes indicating the heart health status of the patients. The categorical data is normalized and represented in the dataset. This chapter aims to predict the risk of a heart attack using three machine learning algorithms. Since both datasets used in this chapter have labeled data, these algorithms should fall under the category of supervised machine learning, where the machine learns from the data provided in the training process to predict the results for the test data. Decision Tree, Random Forest, and K Nearest Neighbors (KNN) are the methods selected for this chapter based on several criteria. Incorporating several datasets permits the identification of issues related to data heterogeneity and sample size limitations and, thereby, the examination of the model's generalizability and reliability.

Keywords: Decision tree, Heart attack, K-Nearest neighbors, Random forest, Supervised machine learning.

INTRODUCTION

Machine learning plays a significant role in diagnosing various medical diseases. Predictive capabilities can impact the health care experience for professionals in early diagnoses and detection, implying prevention strategies and saving lives through early intervention [1]. Nowadays, heart disease statistics according to the American Heart Association, declared in the National Institute of Health in their

* **Corresponding author Abdelhameed Ibrahim:** Faculty of Engineering, Design and Information & Communications Technology (EDICT), School of ICT, Bahrain Polytechnic, PO Box 33349, Isa Town, Bahrain;
E-mail: abdelhameed.fawzy@polytechnic.bh

Neeraj Gupta, Abdelhameed Ibrahim, Bhavesh Vyas & Shobhna Jeet (Eds.)

annual report the impact of some factors like cholesterol, blood pressure, glucose measures, and lifestyle on the possibility of encountering a heart attack [2].

Therefore, this chapter focuses on solving the problem of analyzing the factors that usually trigger heart attacks. It implements supervised machine learning algorithms on two datasets to predict heart attacks through training on data about both the individuals who have experienced heart attacks and those who have not. The symptoms are taken as features to predict whether the patient is at risk of a heart attack and classify new data points. The goal of this chapter is to predict the risk of a heart attack using three machine learning algorithms. Since both datasets used in this chapter have labeled data, these algorithms should fall under the supervised machine learning category, where the machine learns from the provided data in a training process to predict the test data output. K Nearest Neighbors (KNN), Decision Tree, and Random Forest [3] are the methods selected for this chapter based on several criteria that will be explained further.

Machine Learning (ML) can play an essential role in discovering medical risk factors using data-driven methods [4 - 7]. In this chapter, the techniques of machine learning are employed to create predictive models that can effectively diagnose whether patients are having a heart attack or not. The methodology followed to complete the chapter involved gathering real datasets that contain patients' demographic information, medical health factors, and clinical test results. The data is then processed and cleaned to be in suitable formats for the machine learning models training. Moreover, feature selection and scaling techniques were applied to conclude the most relevant predictors of heart attack risk. Afterward, three predictive models, random forest, decision tree, and KNN, were trained on the prepared data to learn the relationships between the features selected and the targeted variable. The method's performance on the created test subset was measured using a variety of metrics, including Mean Square Error (MSE), accuracy, classification report, and confusion matrix. This chapter aimed to provide healthcare practitioners with a predictive model that would identify the heart attack risk for patients to enable them to take early intervention or preventive measures.

The data collection process in this chapter has some associated limitations, as the effectiveness of the ML model relies significantly on the quality and quantity of the data given to train the models. Medical data collection is challenging and raises several ethical and legal considerations, including patients' privacy and data security. Several datasets were tested in this chapter based on the data appropriateness to extract features and train models.

A good data set with only 303 records was found at a point in the data collection process. The quality of data features was excellent for the prediction process; however, the number of records in the data was small. To address this limitation in the number of records, data augmentation was used through repetition, which might exacerbate the overfitting risk. This might lead the ML model to memorize the duplicated instances rather than capturing the patterns. Furthermore, data augmentation was also needed in the second dataset collected because of the significant class imbalance that can occur in the data. Therefore, the Synthetic Minority Over-Sampling Technique (SMOTE) was employed to generate synthetic records based on the features of the minority class samples for class balancing.

MACHINE LEARNING MODELS

Decision Tree (DT) is considered a non-parametric ML algorithm that follows the method of "divide and rule," where the workspace is split into divisions. The DT algorithm uses the principles of greedy search to identify the optimal split points within a search tree. The decision tree structure is like a flowchart, in which the information gained from the dataset increasingly helps in building the tree recursively [8, 9].

The DT method can be utilized well for classification tasks, especially in the medical field, for diagnosing many diseases. Therefore, it is used due to the labeled data, which qualifies this chapter's tasks as classification. This chapter uses the decision tree to classify the labels as zeros or ones according to the given features. The root node is selected based on the highest information gain feature. It splits the tested dataset into many subsets that will be divided recurrently until no more subsets are separated by forming a termination node indicating the end of data [10]. The most important feature of this method is that it can manage the non-linearity in the data (between the features and the heart attack risk) that might sometimes be present in complex medical data. Because of the dataset division, there is no restraint in the relationship between the input variables and labels. This method also has low computational complexity, which makes it suitable for non-large datasets.

The Random Forest (RF) method is commonly employed for regression and classification problems. RF can be considered a bagging method extension that employs feature randomness for an uncorrelated forest of decision trees. The main significant difference between the RF and the decision tree method is that decision trees consider all the possible features for the node split. In contrast, the random forest only selects the subsets of those features to generate decisions. This method was used because it is highly stable. It gives the average answer given by several trees. It does not consider all the features while making each decision tree, which maintains diversity, especially when looking into medical classification tasks. This method efficiently handles binary, continuous, and categorical data [9, 11].

The K-nearest Neighbor method is mainly based on the idea that similar values (labels) tend to similar data points. KNN is suitable for classification and regression tasks because it stores the entire dataset as a reference during training. Within the KNN method, the distance between the input data point and the training samples is calculated using the metric of Euclidean distance during the prediction process. The algorithm then uses the number of input data point's nearest neighbors based on the calculated distance. This chapter investigates the classification tasks where the algorithm for the most common label within the k neighbors is assigned to the input data point. This method is straightforward, but its performance relies significantly on choosing k [12, 13].

EXPERIMENTS

Dataset Selection

This chapter uses two datasets to predict heart attacks, which provides valuable insights into the machine learning algorithms used in the prediction process, as shown in Table **1**. Incorporating several datasets permits the identification of issues related to data heterogeneity and sample size limitations and, thereby, the examination of the model's generalizability and reliability.

Table 1. Dataset details [14, 15].

Dataset Name	Year	Attributes	Type	Dataset Ref.
Heart Attack Analysis & Prediction Dataset(heart.csv)	2021	14	CSV	[14]
Heart attack datasets (Medicaldataset.csv)	2019	9	CSV	[15]

First Dataset

The first dataset used in this chapter is the heart attack risk prediction dataset, which has 14 attributes relevant to heart health, including demographic information of the patient, clinical features, diagnostic test results, symptoms, and risk factors, as well as outcome variables, as shown in Table **2**.

Table 2. First dataset description [14].

Attribute	Data type	Description	Feature
Age	int64	Patient's age	Yes
Sex	int64	Patient's Sex (0: Female / 1: Male)	Yes
Cp	int64	Type of Chest pain: (1: typical anginal / 2: atypical anginal / 3: non-anginal/ 4: asymptomatic)	Yes
trestbps	int64	T resting blood pressure (on admission)	Yes
Chol	int64	Value of the cholesterol level of the patient	Yes
fbs	int64	Boolean of fasting blood sugar (0: False /1: True)	No
restecg	int64	Boolean of resting electrocardiographic (0: normal /1: having ST-T wave abnormality	Yes
Thalachh	int64	Max achieved heart rate	Yes
Exng	int64	Boolean of exercise-induced angina. (0: No / 1: Yes)	Yes
Oldpeak	float64	ST depression induced	No
Slp	Int64	Peak exercise ST segment slope (0: down sloping/ 1: flat/ 2: upsloping)	Yes
caa	int64	Major vessels number (0–3)	No
thall	int64	Blood disorder called thalassemia value (1: fixed defect / 2: normal blood flow/3: reversible defect)	No
output	int64	Boolean of heart attack presence (0: No / 1: Yes)	No

This data frame contains 303 records and 14 columns with a total memory usage of 33.3 KB. Each row in the dataset is a distinct observation for a different patient. The datatypes of the columns in this data frame are integers and floats, denoting the different attributes associated with each observation record by a mixture of both numerical and categorical features. This dataset was cleaned and contains no null values; however, it is a small dataset because of the number of records, which is correspondingly little for the use of machine learning methods. The need for data augmentation is urgent and crucial to enhance the dataset's size and diversity for effective machine learning.

The dataset has one duplicated record removed before augmenting the data for the ML algorithm to generalize on the unseen data. That is because of the violation assumption that the sample duplication will commonly be deployed on the machine learning model with varying effects, as they will not offer new knowledge to the model [16]. Although this project uses data repetition to augment the data frame with new records, it is essential to remove these duplicated records to eliminate any chance of bias or noise in the augmented dataset.

The method used for augmenting the data frame with new data involves repeating the original data to reach the desired length of the data frame. While this increases the variety of available samples for training the model, it also has potential drawbacks. Simply repeating the data may mislead the model, making it unable to generalize precisely on new data. To mitigate this, the method introduces some level of randomness and variation to the augmented dataset by adding carefully controlled random fractions of the original dataset.

The descriptive statistics were generated using Pandas' library, which provides valuable insights into the numerical columns in the data frame, their distributions, and potential outliers.

- The **count** record shows the number of non-null values in the columns. Each column has 600 records, which means that the data frame has no null values.
- **Mean** shows the average value of the columns in this data frame, with the following insights:
- Age: the average age of the patient in the data frame is 54.37 years old.
- Sex: the proportion of males is higher in this data frame, as shown by the mean of the sex column: 0.68, where (0: female /1: male).
- Trtbps: shows the mean value of 131.62 mm/Hg for the resting blood pressure.
- Chol: the mean value 246.26 mg/dl of the cholesterol level in the data frame.
- Fbs: the mean value of the fasting blood sugar of 0.15 represents the proportion of patients with blood sugar in fasting higher than 20 mg/dl.
- Thalachh: the mean maximum heart rate is 149.65.
- Exng: the mean value of exercise-induced angina is 0.33, which represents the proportion of patients with the symptom.
- Output: the mean value of patients' heart attack in the data frame is 0.54.
- **Standard Deviation (Std)** measures the spread of values around the mean, where a higher std means a higher variability of data in the column.
- **Min** shows the minimum **values** in the columns:
- Age: the minimum age in the dataset is 29.
- Trtbps: the minimum resting blood pressure in the dataset is 94mm/Hg.
- Chol: the minimum cholesterol level in the dataset is 126 mg/dl.
- Thalachh: the minimum of the maximum heart rate achieved is 71 beats per minute.
- **Max** shows the **maximum** values in the columns:
- Age: the maximum age in the dataset is 77.
- Trtbps: the maximum value of resting blood pressure in the dataset is 200mm/Hg.
- Chol: the maximum value of the cholesterol level in the dataset is 564 mg/dl.

- Thalachh: the maximum of the maximum heart rate achieved is 202 beats per minute.
- **25% - 50% - 75%** indicators show the first quartile, median and third quartile of the data percentile in each column.

Fig. (**1**) shows the heart attack risk class distribution in the first data frame. The initially used dataset had 165 records with the incidence of a heart attack and 138 records without heart attack. After augmenting the data with synthetic data, the number of samples in the dataset belonging to each class has changed to 326 records with the incidence of a heart attack and 274 records without a heart attack. The data is reasonably but not perfectly balanced, as there is an approximately equal distribution of both classes, with the same ratio of 1.19 for both data frames, where the heart attack incidence is 0.19 more than the class with no incidence of a heart attack.

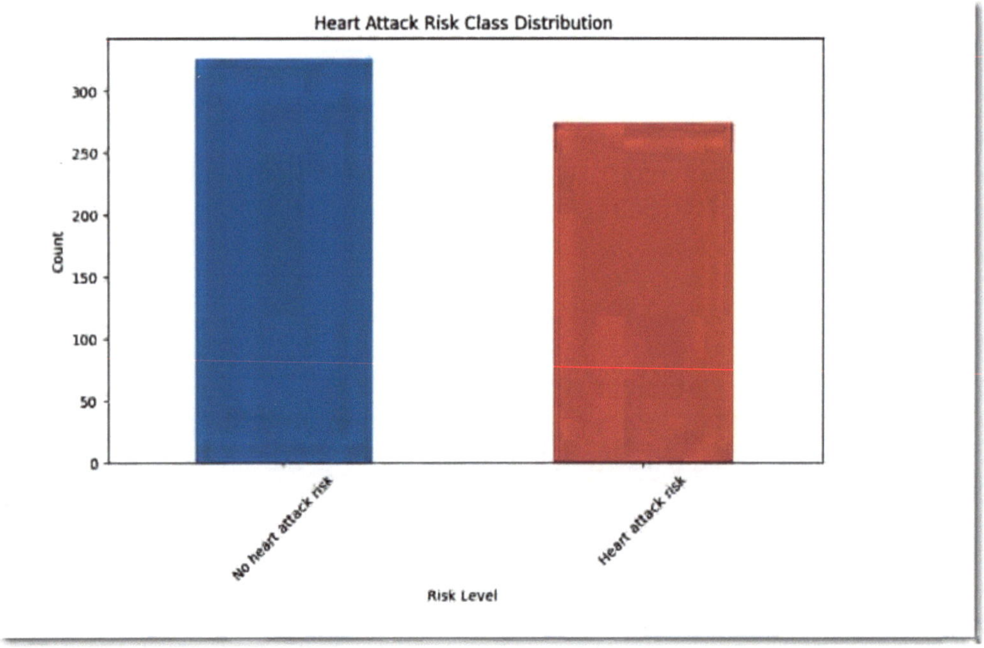

Fig. (1). Heart attack risk class distribution in the first data frame.

The class distribution of gender in the dataset shows that males have more samples than females, with male samples representing approximately 68% of the data (409 samples) and female samples representing approximately 32% of the data (191 samples).

The class distribution of the age shows a diverse age of patients with the spectrum range between 29 and 77. This wide age range presents an intriguing opportunity to explore potential correlations between age and heart attack occurrence. A notable concentration of patients in this dataset shows in the mid-range of ages between 40 and 60 years old.

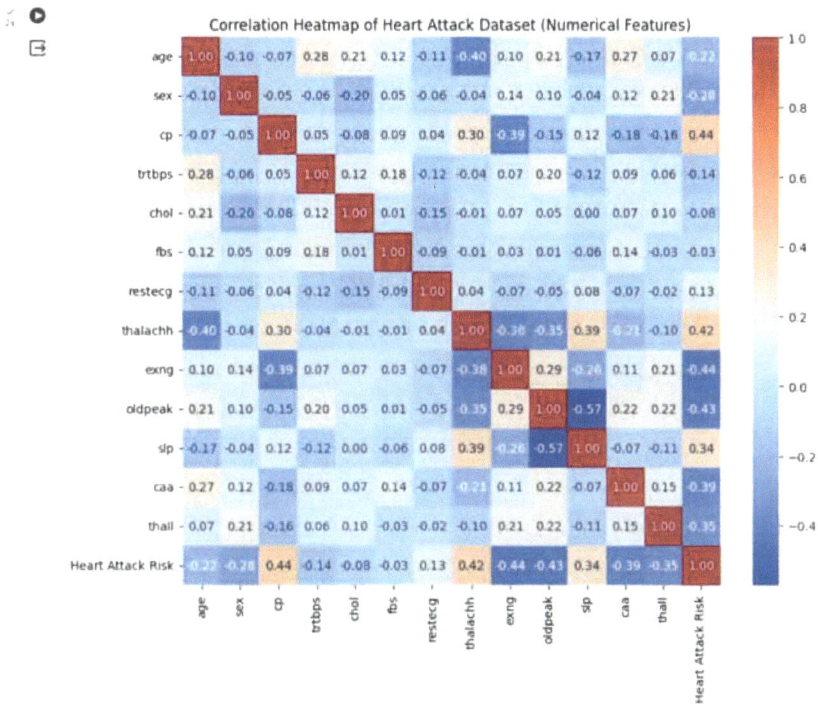

Fig. (2). First data frame attributes correlation map: Heart attack risk correlation with other features.

The heat map in Fig. (**2**) shows a correlation map of a heart attack for various attributes in the dataset; the heart attack risk correlates with the maximum heart rate (Thalach), chest pain type(CP), and the slope of the peak exercise ST segment (slp) moderately. It also correlates negatively with the number of major vessels (CAA), exercise-induced angina (EX-Angina), ST depression induced by exercise relative to rest (Old Peak), and thalassemia (thal). In addition, heart attack risk has a low correlation with age, sex, and resting electrocardiographic results (restECG). These correlations insinuate that specific attributes may indicate whether the risk of a heart attack will increase or decrease.

Second Dataset

The second dataset used in this chapter is the heart attack dataset (Medicaldataset.csv). It was collected in Iraq at Zheen Hospital in Erbil in 2019. The dataset has 1319 records of patients and nine attributes indicating their heart health status. The categorical data is normalized and represented in the dataset, as shown in Table **3**.

Table 3. Second dataset description [15].

Attribute	Data type	Description	Feature
Age	int64	Patient's age	Yes
Gender	int64	Patient's gender (0: Female / 1: Male)	Yes
Heart rate	int64	Heart rate of the patient	Yes
Systolic blood pressure	int64	The pressure measure in the arteries when the heart beats.	Yes
Diastolic blood pressure	int64	The pressure measure in the arteries when the heart rests between beats.	Yes
Blood sugar	float64	Level of fasting blood sugar	No
CK-MB	float64	Level of a creatine kinase-myocardial band enzyme in blood.	Yes
Troponin	float64	The level of the troponin protein in the blood.	Yes
Result	object	Presence of heart attack (Negative/Positive)	No(target)

The data frame contains 1319 non-null records and 9 columns, using approximately 93 KB of memory. Each row in the dataset is a distinct observation for a different patient. The datatypes of columns in this data frame are integers and floats, denoting the different attributes associated with each observation record by numerical and categorical features. The target column datatype is an object that contains string values that need to be converted into numerical values.

This data frame is unique in that it does not contain any duplicated values. The descriptive statistics, which provide valuable insights about the numerical columns in the data frame, are particularly noteworthy.

- The count record shows the number of non-null values in the columns. Each column has 1319 records, which means that the data frame has no null values.
- **Mean** shows the average value of the columns in this data frame, with the following insights:
    - Age: the average age of the patient in the data frame is 56.19 years old.
    - Gender: the proportion of males is higher in this data frame, as shown by the

mean of the sex column: 0.65, where (0: female /1: male).
   - Heart rate: shows the mean value of 78.33 beats per minute.
   - Systolic blood pressure: mean blood pressure value is 127.17 mm/Hg.
   - Diastolic blood pressure: resting blood pressure mean value is 72.26 mm/Hg.
   - Blood sugar: the mean blood sugar value is 74.9 mg/dl.
   - CK-MB: the mean level of a creatine kinase-myocardial band enzyme in the blood is 15.7.
   - Troponin: the mean value of the level of troponin protein in the blood is 0.36.
- **Min** shows the minimum values in the columns:
   - Age: the minimum age in the dataset is 14.
   - Heart rate: the minimum heart rate is 20.
   - Systolic blood pressure: the minimum blood pressure in the dataset is 42mm/Hg.
   - Diastolic blood pressure: the minimum resting blood pressure in the dataset is 38 mm/Hg.
   - Blood sugar: the minimum blood sugar level in the dataset is 35 mg/dl.
   - CK-MB: the minimum creatine kinase-myocardial band enzyme in the blood is 0.321.
   - Troponin: thc minimum Troponin level is 0.001.
- **Max** shows the maximum values in the columns:
   - Age: the maximum age in the dataset is 103.
   - Heart rate: the maximum heart rate is 111.
   - Systolic blood pressure: the maximum blood pressure in the dataset is 223 mm/Hg.
   - Diastolic blood pressure: the maximum resting blood pressure in the dataset is 154 mm/Hg.
   - Blood sugar: the maximum blood sugar level in the dataset is 541 mg/dl.
   - CK-MB: the maximum creatine kinase-myocardial band enzyme in the blood is 300.
   - Troponin: the maximum Troponin level is 10.3.

The distribution in Fig. (**3**) clearly shows the data imbalance in the data frame between the two classes (presence of heart attack risk / no heart attack risk). The positive class has significantly more instances than the negative. There are 810 records with a positive heart attack presence and 509 records without. This problem can be addressed by methods based on oversampling or downsampling, such as SMOTE, ADASYN, and RUS, *etc* [17].

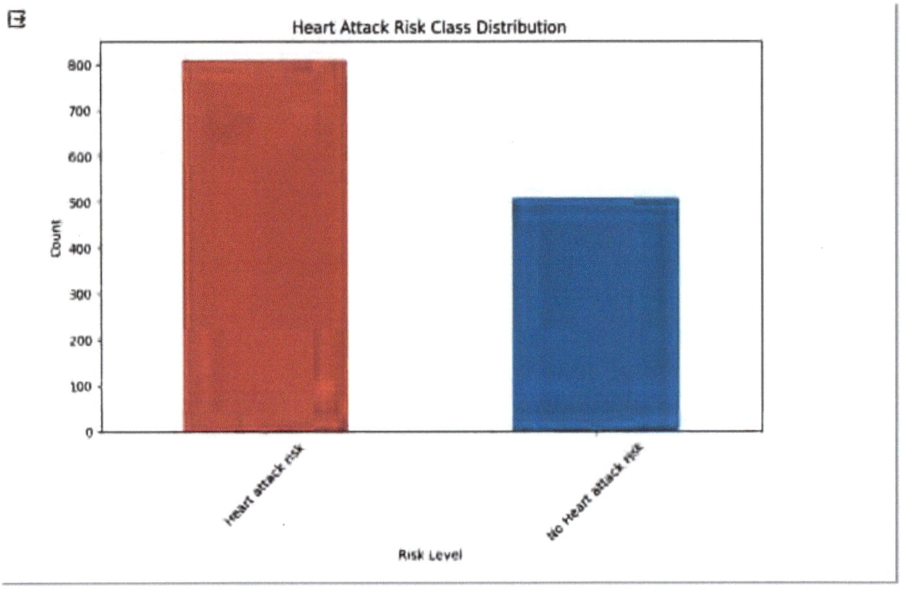

Fig. (3). Heart attack risk class distribution in the second data frame.

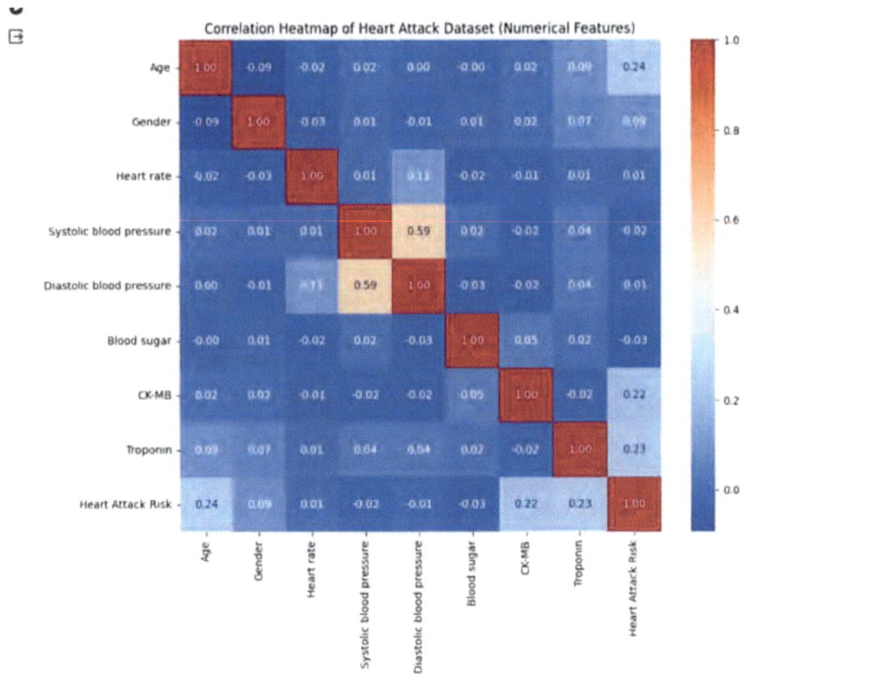

Fig. (4). Second data frame attributes correlation map.

The heat map in Fig. (**4**) shows a correlation map for heart attack based on various attributes in the dataset; the risk of heart attack correlates with age, CK-MB, and Troponin moderately, indicating a more substantial relationship than other attributes in the data frame.

Preparing the Data

In the first data preparation process, the target variable 'Heart attack risk was separated from the features set to ensure that the target variable was not used in the features for training the model, and then dataset was split into training and testing subsets by the 'train_test_split" function ensuring that 80% is used for training the model and 20% for testing it with a random state value of 1. The numerical features are scaled to remove the mean from the data, and the scaler was fitted to both the training and the testing subsets.

For the second dataset, the features were also separated from the target, and then the features were scaled using the standard scaler. Moreover, since the data classes are imbalanced, the SMOTE Technique was used to balance the classes by increasing the minority class. The data is then split into training and testing subsets, with proportions of 80% for the training process and 20% for the testing, using a random state value of 1.

The Performance of Machine Learning Methods

The performance metrics employed in this evaluation are accuracy, Mean Squares Error (MSE), and Root Mean Square Error (RMSE) [18 - 21]. Table **4** shows the models' performance on the first dataset. Based on the metrics evaluation of the methods used on the first datasets, Random Forest appears to have the highest accuracy on the dataset (0.925), the lowest MSE (0.075), and the lowest RMSE (0.273). Therefore, it is the best method performed on this dataset as it demonstrates superior performance in classifying the data compared to the other models. Fig. (**5**) presents the Random Forest performance chart on the first dataset. Fig. (**6**) shows the Random Forest prediction numbers on the first test data.

Table 4. Models' performance on the first dataset.

Model	Accuracy	Mse	Rmse
Decision Tree	0.9	0.1	0.316
Random Forest	0.925	0.075	0.273
K-Nearest Neighbor	0.875	0.125	0.353

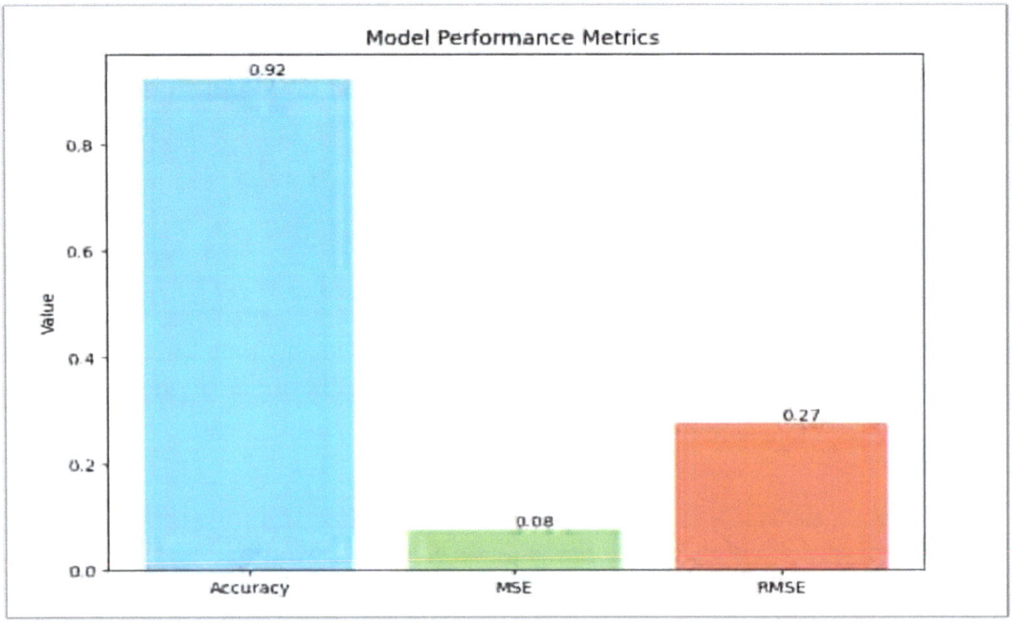

Fig. (5). Random forest performance chart on the first dataset.

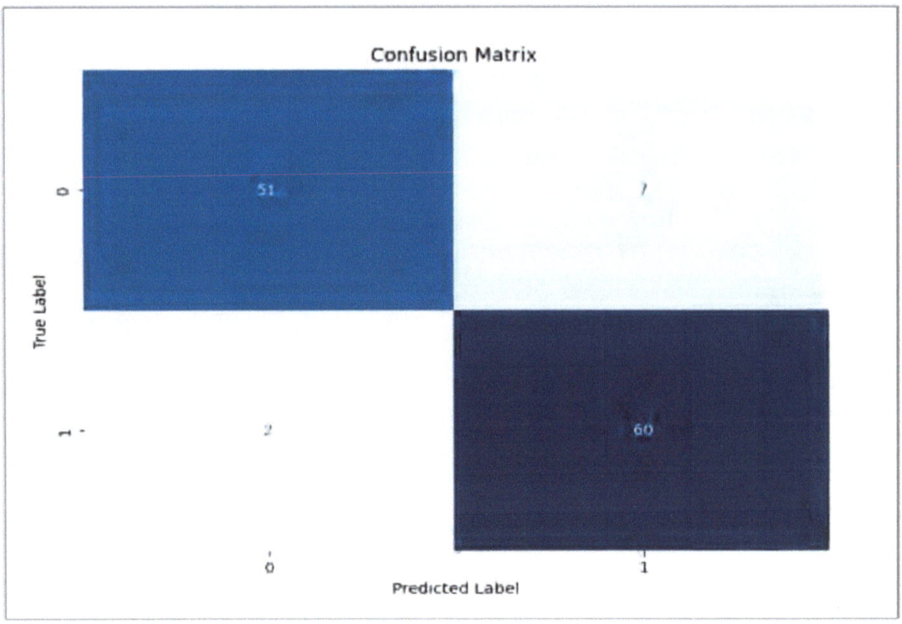

Fig. (6). Random forest prediction numbers on the first test data

Table **5** shows the models' performance on the second dataset. Both the decision tree and the random forest models perform the same for the second dataset. Both models have achieved a high accuracy of 98.7% and low MSE and RMSE rates of 0.0123 and 0.111. This indicates that the models perform exceptionally well in data classification with minimal errors. By showcasing the models' performance on the test data, insight into how the model generalizes on unseen data is captured, which indicates its reliability in practical applications. Fig. (**7**) presents the performance chart for the Decision Tree and Random Forest on the second dataset. Fig. (**8**) shows the Decision tree and Random Forest prediction numbers on the second test data.

Table 5. Models' performance on the second dataset.

MODEL	Accuracy	MSE	RMSE
Decision Tree	0.987	0.0123	0.111
Random Forest	0.987	0.0123	0.111
K Nearest Neighbor	0.663	0.336	0.58

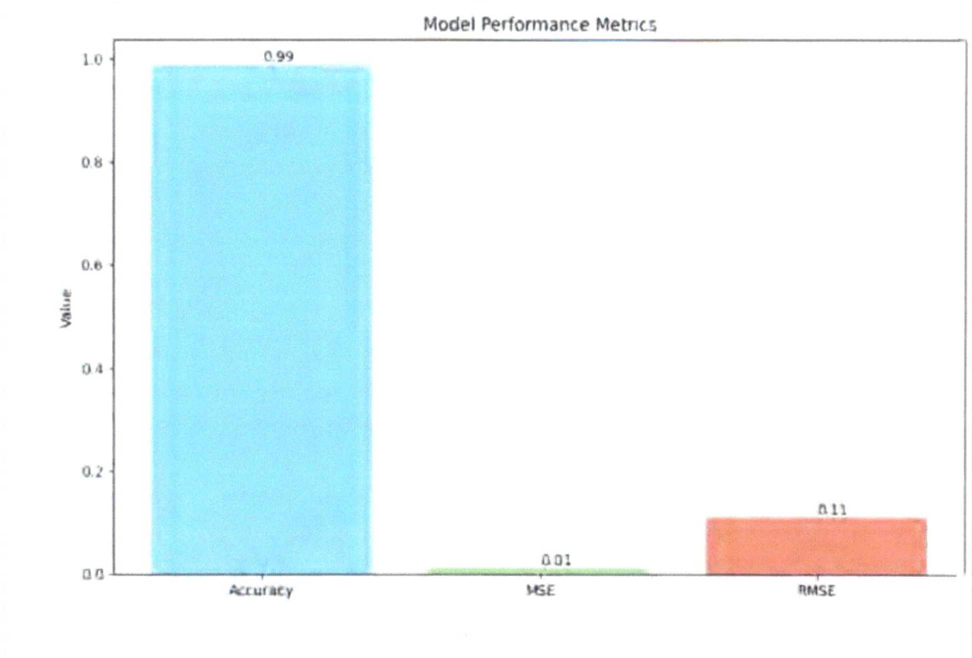

Fig. (7). Decision tree and Random Forest performance chart on the second dataset.

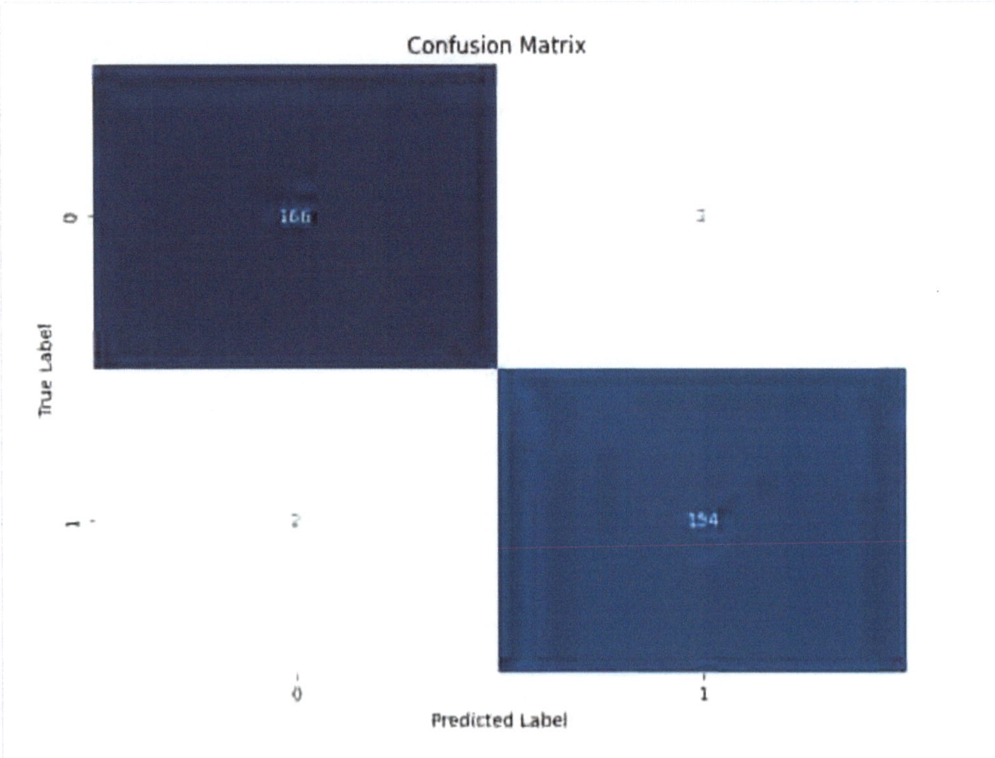

Fig. (8). Decision tree and Random Forest prediction numbers on the second test data.

CONCLUDING REMARKS

While clinical methods can successfully predict heart attacks, technology can contribute significantly and help in identifying heart attacks. Machine learning can provide accurate and reliable predictive algorithms that unveil medical data patterns. Several supervised learning algorithms can apply regression and classification tasks to medical data, such as the Bayesian algorithm and the support vector machine algorithm SVM, among many more. Conversely, in this chapter, three powerful machine-learning algorithms were used to create classifiers with feature selections. The highest accuracy was achieved by the random forest algorithm, with values of 0.925 on the first dataset and 0.987 on the second dataset, indicating the machine learning method's ability to accurately predict heart attacks using essential patient data, rather than relying on costly ECG scans. Machine learning may offer significant advancements in the medical field, particularly in diagnosing various diseases based on patient input.

For future work, several data augmentation techniques will be combined to handle the imbalance of classes in the medical datasets such as SMOTE, as explained before, Under-sampling (US), which reduces the samples in the majority class, Particle Swarm Optimization (PSO) for tuning the parameters of SMOTE, and Meta Cost which adjust the decision threshold of the classifier based on the classification problem. Integrating the three techniques mitigates their limitations, creating a more balanced and representative dataset to train the classifiers [22]. In addition, in future work, the chapter can extract the results of the prediction process into a CSV file to explore the machine learning algorithms' predictions and compare the results with the actual data. The CSV output can also be enhanced to contain additional information, such as probabilities or confidence scores associated with each predicted class for each prediction.

REFERENCES

[1] Tsao, C. W., Aday, A. W., Almarzooq, Z. I., *et al.* (2023, February 21). Heart Disease and Stroke Statistics—2023 Update: A Report From the American Heart Association. Circulation, e93-e621. Available from: https://www.ahajournals.org/doi/10.1161/CIR.0000000000001123

[2] Gavhane A, Kokkula G, Pandya I, Devadkar K. Prediction of heart disease using machine learning. Second international conference on electronics, communication and aerospace technology 2018; 1275-8.
[http://dx.doi.org/10.1109/ICECA.2018.8474922]

[3] El-kenawy ESM, Mirjalili S, Khodadadi N, *et al.* Feature selection in wind speed forecasting systems based on meta-heuristic optimization. PLoS One 2023; 18(2): e0278491.
[http://dx.doi.org/10.1371/journal.pone.0278491] [PMID: 36749744]

[4] Alhussan AA, Abdelhamid AA, Towfek SK, *et al.* Classification of diabetes using feature selection and hybrid al-biruni earth radius and dipper throated optimization. Diagnostics (Basel) 2023; 13(12): 2038.
[http://dx.doi.org/10.3390/diagnostics13122038] [PMID: 37370932]

[5] Alharbi AH, Towfek SK, Abdelhamid AA, *et al.* Diagnosis of monkeypox disease using transfer learning and binary advanced dipper throated optimization algorithm. Biomimetics (Basel) 2023; 8(3): 313.
[http://dx.doi.org/10.3390/biomimetics8030313] [PMID: 37504202]

[6] Eid MM, El-Kenawy ESM, Khodadadi N, *et al.* Meta-heuristic optimization of LSTM-based deep network for boosting the prediction of monkeypox cases. Mathematics 2022; 10(20): 3845.
[http://dx.doi.org/10.3390/math10203845]

[7] Atteia G, Abdel Samee N, El-Kenawy ESM, Ibrahim A. CNN-hyperparameter optimization for diabetic maculopathy diagnosis in optical coherence tomography and fundus retinography. Mathematics 2022; 10(18): 3274.
[http://dx.doi.org/10.3390/math10183274]

[8] IBM. (n.d.). What is a decision tree? From IBM: Available from: https://www.ibm.com/topics/decision-trees

[9] El-Sayed M. El-kenawy, Abdelhameed Ibrahim, *et al.* Optimized Ensemble Algorithm for Predicting Metamaterial Antenna Parameters, Computers. Materials & Continua 2022; 71(3): 4989-5003.
[http://dx.doi.org/10.32604/cmc.2022.023884]

[10] Mineni H. Second heart attack prediction using machine learning and deep learning. Dublin: Dublin Business School 2020.

[11] IBM. (n.d.). What is random forest? From IBM: Available from: https://www.ibm.com/topics/random-forest

[12] El-Kenawy ESM, Khodadadi N, Mirjalili S, *et al.* Metaheuristic optimization for improving weed detection in wheat images captured by drones. Mathematics 2022; 10(23): 4421. [http://dx.doi.org/10.3390/math10234421]

[13] Shams MY, Elshewey AM, El-kenawy ESM, Ibrahim A, Talaat FM, Tarek Z. Water quality prediction using machine learning models based on grid search method. Multimedia Tools Appl 2023; 83(12): 35307-34. [http://dx.doi.org/10.1007/s11042-023-16737-4]

[14] Heart Disease, https://archive.ics.uci.edu/dataset/45/heart+disease, Last visited 1-08-2024.

[15] Heart Attack Dataset, https://data.mendeley.com/datasets/wmhctcrt5v/1, Last visited 1-08-2024.

[16] Zhao Y, Li L, Wang H, *et al.* On the impact of sample duplication in machine-learning-based android malware detection. ACM Trans Softw Eng Methodol 2021; 30(3): 1-38. [http://dx.doi.org/10.1145/3446905]

[17] Viloria A, Pineda Lezama OB, Mercado-Caruzo N. Unbalanced data processing using oversampling: Machine Learning. Procedia Comput Sci. 2020;175:108-113. [http://dx.doi.org/10.1016/j.procs.2020.07.018]

[18] Djaafari A, Ibrahim A, Bailek N, *et al.* Hourly predictions of direct normal irradiation using an innovative hybrid LSTM model for concentrating solar power projects in hyper-arid regions. Energy Rep 2022; 8: 15548-62. [http://dx.doi.org/10.1016/j.egyr.2022.10.402]

[19] El-Sayed M. El-kenawy, Abdelaziz A. Abdelhamid, Abdelhameed Ibrahim, *et al.* Al-Biruni Earth Radius (BER) metaheuristic search optimization algorithm. Comput Syst Sci Eng 2023; 45(2): 1917-34. [http://dx.doi.org/10.32604/csse.2023.032497]

[20] Khafaga DS, Ibrahim A, El-Kenawy ESM, *et al.* An al-biruni earth radius optimization-based deep convolutional neural network for classifying monkeypox disease. Diagnostics (Basel) 2022; 12(11): 2892. [http://dx.doi.org/10.3390/diagnostics12112892] [PMID: 36428952]

[21] El-Kenawy EM, Zerouali B, Bailek N, *et al.* Improved weighted ensemble learning for predicting the daily reference evapotranspiration under the semi-arid climate conditions. Environ Sci Pollut Res Int 2022; 29(54): 81279-99. [http://dx.doi.org/10.1007/s11356-022-21410-8] [PMID: 35731435]

[22] Wang YC, Cheng CH. A multiple combined method for rebalancing medical data with class imbalances. Comput Biol Med 2021; 134: 104527. [http://dx.doi.org/10.1016/j.compbiomed.2021.104527] [PMID: 34091384]

CHAPTER 7

Predictive Analysis of Cardiovascular Health Through Machine Learning

Bedour Aldalbahi[1] and **Abdelhameed Ibrahim**[1,*]

[1] *School of ICT, Faculty of Engineering, Design and Information & Communications Technology (EDICT), Bahrain Polytechnic, PO Box 33349, Isa Town, Bahrain*

Abstract: Cardiovascular illnesses are a significant contributor to illness and death on a global scale, highlighting the importance of identifying them early and implementing preventative healthcare measures. The highest heart rate reached during physical activity, referred to as 'heartRate', is a crucial measure of an individual's cardiovascular well-being. Precisely forecasting this parameter can aid in promptly identifying individuals in danger, enabling immediate medical intervention. This study uses machine learning techniques to forecast 'heartRate' by examining various physiological and clinical characteristics. The chapter describes the utilization of Linear Regression, Random Forest, and Gradient Boosting models, with each model evaluated for its prediction accuracy. This work examines the inherent obstacles in machine learning applications in healthcare, including data imbalance and model interpretability. It offers a thorough review of the effectiveness of models used for predicting cardiovascular health indicators. This undertaking is not solely focused on forecasting a numerical value but on comprehending the complex connections among many health variables and how they collectively impact cardiovascular function. The goal is to aid in the early diagnosis of health issues and provide individualized healthcare solutions.

Keywords: Cardiovascular health, Gradient boosting regressor, Linear regression, Machine learning, Predictive analysis.

INTRODUCTION

The chapter explores the domain of predictive healthcare, explicitly examining the estimation of the maximum heart rate attainable during physical exercise, which is a crucial indicator of cardiovascular well-being. Using Machine Learning (ML) methods, the research intends to forecast the heart rate by analyzing a wide range of physiological and clinical characteristics [1, 2]. This would help in detecting potential heart-related health issues at an early stage. The main goal is to employ

* **Corresponding author Abdelhameed Ibrahim:** School of ICT, Faculty of Engineering, Design and Information & Communications Technology (EDICT), Bahrain Polytechnic, PO Box 33349, Isa Town, Bahrain;
E-mail: abdelhameed.fawzy@polytechnic.bh

Neeraj Gupta, Abdelhameed Ibrahim, Bhavesh Vyas & Shobhna Jeet (Eds.)

machine learning techniques to effectively estimate and predict the heart rate. This undertaking is not solely focused on forecasting a numerical value, but on comprehending the complex connections among many health variables and how they collectively impact cardiovascular function. The main objective is to develop a tool that can assist healthcare providers in proactively identifying patients with an elevated susceptibility to cardiovascular illnesses.

This chapter examines the utilization of ML methods to forecast the maximum attainable heart rate in individuals, a vital measure for evaluating cardiovascular well-being. Machine learning can play an important role in discovering medical risk factors using data-driven methods [3, 4]. The study uses three major machine learning models, Regressor of Random Forest Linear Regression [5 - 7], and Regressor of Gradient Boosting [8], to analyze physiological and clinical characteristics. The metrics of R-squared (R^2), Mean Absolute Error (MAE), and Mean Squared Error (MSE) [9 - 12] are used to assess the performance of each model on the tested dataset.

The chapter addresses obstacles such as imbalanced data, high dimensionality, and processing limitations to enhance the accuracy of the employed models. The results illustrate the considerable capacity of ML to improve the accuracy of predictions and provide valuable information for assessing cardiovascular health in the tested dataset. The goal is to aid in the early diagnosis of health issues and provide individualized healthcare solutions. This can facilitate early detection of heart disease, improving treatment outcomes. It can also optimize healthcare resource allocation by identifying high-risk individuals and advance research in applying machine learning to healthcare diagnostics.

PROBLEM DESCRIPTION

This chapter aims at leveraging Machine Learning (ML) to predict the maximum heart rate achieved (thalach) by individuals, which is a critical measure in assessing heart disease risk. By analyzing various physiological and clinical features alongside 'thalach', the chapter seeks to enable the early identification of individuals at risk for heart disease, potentially facilitating timely intervention and management.

MACHINE LEARNING LIBRARIES

The following libraries will be employed in this work [13].

- The pandas package is applied for data manipulation and ingestion.
- The Numpy package is applied for numerical operations.

- The Matplotlib.pyplot and Seaborn packages are used to visualize the data, facilitating an understanding of the distributions of various features and the target variable.
- **Sklearn** is used for its comprehensive suite of tools for machine learning, including various machine learning models that are imported for building predictive models.
- StandardScaler and MinMaxScaler are applied for feature scaling to normalize the tested dataset and improve the model training.

DATASET DESCRIPTION AND DATA PROCESSING

Dataset Description

The heart disease dataset encompasses a broad array of physiological and clinical features associated with heart disease. The dataset provides a comprehensive overview of patients' characteristics and their correlation with heart disease, with 1027 entries [14]. The features include:

- **Demographic Factors:**
  - Age: Patient's age.
  - Sex (female or male).
- **Behavioral Factors:**
  - Cp (Chest Pain Type): Serum cholesterol in mg/dl.
- **Medical History Factors:**
  - Fbs: Fasting blood sugar > 120 mg/dl (false or true).
  - Restecg: Categorizes resting electrocardiographic results into 3 types.
- **Medical Current Conditions:**
  - Trestbps (Resting Blood Pressure)
  - Chol: Serum cholesterol in mg/dl.
  - Thalach: Highest heart rate achieved.
  - Exang: Exercise-induced chest pain (yes or no).
  - Oldpeak: ST depression induced by exercise relative to rest.
  - Slope: peak exercise ST segment slope.
  - Ca: number of major vessels (0-4) colored by fluoroscopy.
  - Thal: thallium stress test results indicating probable heart disease (values 0-3).

Fig. (**1**) shows the dataset statistical information, and Fig. (**2**) presents the dataset correlation analysis.

```
# Displaying statistical information about the dataset
print (Heart_data.describe())

               age          sex           cp     trestbps         chol  \
count  1027.000000  1027.000000  1027.000000  1027.000000  1027.000000
mean     54.411879     0.695229     0.940604   131.530672   245.764362
std       9.144326     0.460535     1.029476    17.595625    51.817785
min      18.000000     0.000000     0.000000    90.000000   125.000000
25%      48.000000     0.000000     0.000000   120.000000   211.000000
50%      56.000000     1.000000     1.000000   130.000000   240.000000
75%      61.000000     1.000000     2.000000   140.000000   275.000000
max      77.000000     1.000000     3.000000   200.000000   564.000000

               fbs      restecg      thalach        exang      oldpeak  \
count  1027.000000  1027.000000  1027.000000  1027.000000  1027.000000
mean      0.148978     0.528724   148.960078     0.335930     1.069426
std       0.356240     0.527880    23.246693     0.472545     1.174858
min       0.000000     0.000000    70.000000     0.000000     0.000000
25%       0.000000     0.000000   132.000000     0.000000     0.000000
50%       0.000000     1.000000   152.000000     0.000000     0.800000
75%       0.000000     1.000000   166.000000     1.000000     1.800000
max       1.000000     2.000000   202.000000     1.000000     6.200000

             slope           ca         thal       target
count  1027.000000  1027.000000  1027.000000  1027.000000
mean      1.382668     0.755599     2.320351     0.513145
std       0.620171     1.032444     0.625642     0.500071
min       0.000000     0.000000     0.000000     0.000000
25%       1.000000     0.000000     2.000000     0.000000
50%       1.000000     0.000000     2.000000     1.000000
75%       2.000000     1.000000     3.000000     1.000000
max       2.000000     4.000000     3.000000     1.000000
```

Fig. (1). Dataset statistical information.

An integral part of our data exploration was to conduct a correlation analysis to assess the relationships between different features and the target variable. The correlation matrix heatmap is a powerful visual tool that illustrates the relationship between each attribute and every other attribute. The values range from -1 to 1, where 0 suggests no correlation.

Key Insights from the Correlation Matrix

- Target Correlation: The 'cp' and 'thalach' show a notable positive correlation with the target variable, suggesting that these features are important indicators for the presence of heart disease.

- Cholesterol Level: Surprisingly, 'chol' (serum cholesterol) has a weak correlation with the target, indicating that higher cholesterol levels are not as strongly associated with heart disease in this dataset as might be expected.
- Age Factor: Age shows a negative correlation with 'thalach' and a positive one with 'oldpeak' (ST depression), which could signify that older patients tend to have lower maximum heart rates and more exercise-induced ST depression.

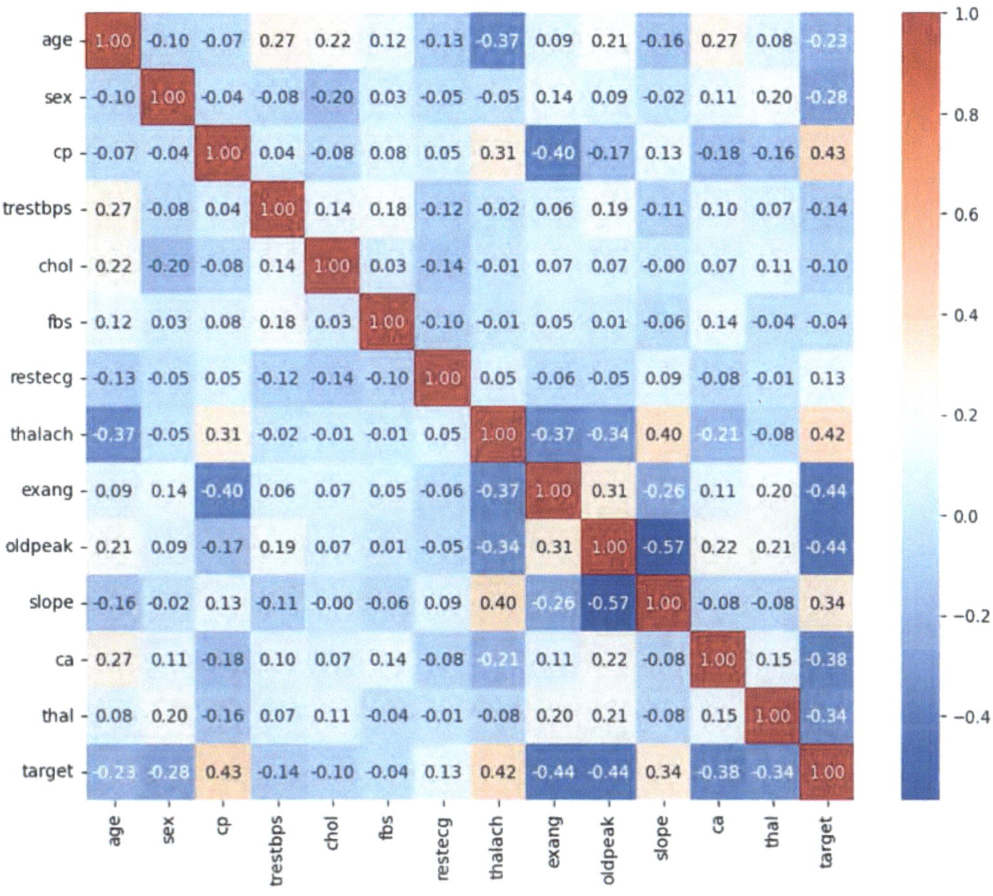

Fig. (2). Dataset correlation analysis.

MACHINE LEARNING MODELS

Linear Regression

The Linear Regression model focuses on the relationship between a scalar response and one or more explanatory variables. This can be achieved by fitting a linear equation to the observed data. The main target of this model is to find a linear combination based on the independent variables that can best predict the dependent variable. Its simplicity and interpretability make Linear Regression an excellent baseline model. It allows for an easy understanding of how each feature impacts the target variable, which is essential for initial exploratory analyses in medical datasets. Default settings were used, with no regularization applied.

Random Forest Regressor

Random Forest is typically trained with the bagging method. The overall prediction is made by averaging the predictions of each component tree. It tends to perform well on a wide range of problems, even without hyperparameter tuning. Chosen for its ability to handle overfitting more effectively than individual Decision Trees, especially in datasets with high dimensionality and complex structures, it is also capable of capturing non-linear relationships between features and the target variable [9, 11]. The parameters will be n_estimators=150, max_features='sqrt', and random_state=42 for reproducibility.

Gradient Boosting Regressor

Gradient Boosting constructs an additive model in which each new tree is built to correct errors made by previously trained trees. It is selected for its precision and effectiveness in various scenarios, including regression and classification problems. The algorithm's strength lies in its ability to reduce both bias and variance in the model by sequentially focusing on instances that are difficult to predict. The parameters will be n_estimators=100, learning_rate=0.05, max_depth=4, and random_state=42.

These algorithms were chosen for their broad applicability and proven track record in predictive modeling, especially in healthcare contexts where the accurate prediction of outcomes, such as heart rate, can directly influence patient treatment plans. The selection of parameters and evaluation of model performance were conducted with careful consideration of both the models' theoretical underpinnings and practical implications, aiming to balance accuracy, complexity, and interpretability in the final predictive modeling solution.

EXPERIMENTS

This section shows the results of application of ML models for the tested dataset. The experimental setup workflow consists of the following steps. The data preprocessing involves normalizing features using MinMaxScaler and splitting the dataset into two sets, with 80% allocated for training and 20% for testing. Training models like Linear Regression and Random Forest Regression uses the training set. Hyperparameters are optimized through grid search or randomized search. MSE, MAE, and R^2 are used to evaluate model performance on the testing set.

The provided scatter plot in Fig. (**3**) shows a comparison of actual *vs.* predicted 'thalach' values. A concentration of points along the diagonal dashed line indicates areas where the model's predictions closely match the actual data. Most data points cluster around the line of identity, suggesting that the model of Linear Regression has a reasonable prediction accuracy. However, there is some scatter away from the line, particularly in the middle range of the actual values, indicating areas where the model's predictions deviate from the true values. The linear regression model demonstrates competence in predicting the maximum heart rate achievable, particularly for values closer to the line of identity. While there are deviations, especially for mid-range heart rates, the model generally captures the trend in the data. Further model diagnostics, such as calculating the residuals and checking for homoscedasticity, would provide more insights into the model's predictive capabilities and areas for improvement.

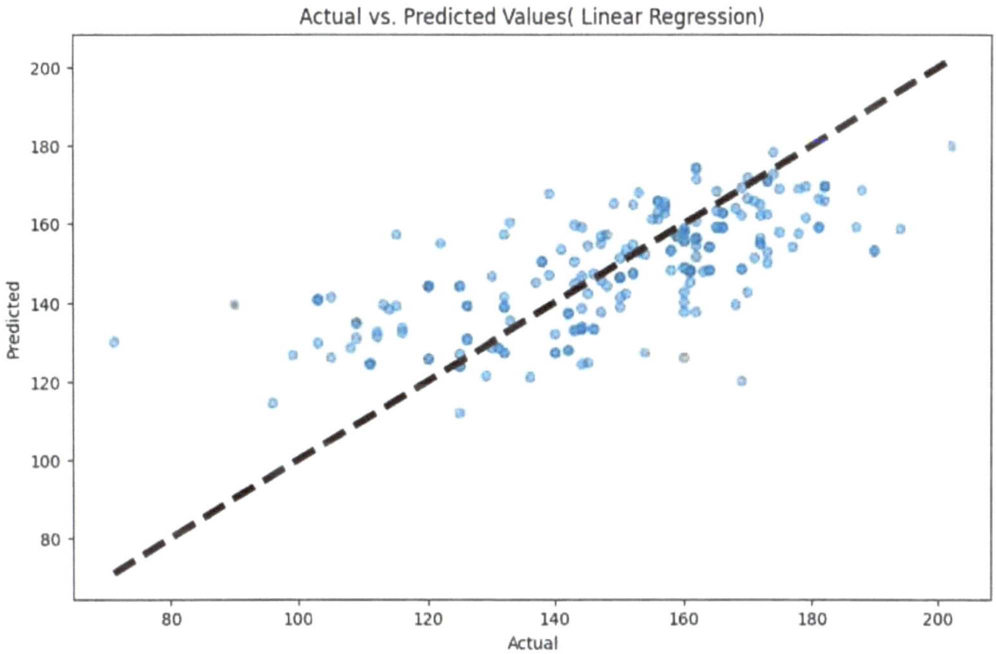

Fig. (3). Linear regression result.

The plot in Fig. (**4**) displays the actual *vs* the predicted 'thalach' values from the Random Forest Regressor, with green dots symbolizing the model's predictions and the dashed line representing the ideal prediction line where actual and predicted values match perfectly. The tight clustering of green dots around the diagonal indicates that the Random Forest Regressor has achieved a high degree of accuracy, with predictions closely aligning with the actual values across the range. The Random Forest Regressor demonstrates robust predictive capabilities, as reflected by the dense grouping of predictions along the line of the perfect fit, suggesting that it can be a reliable tool for estimating 'thalach' in the context of heart disease risk assessment.

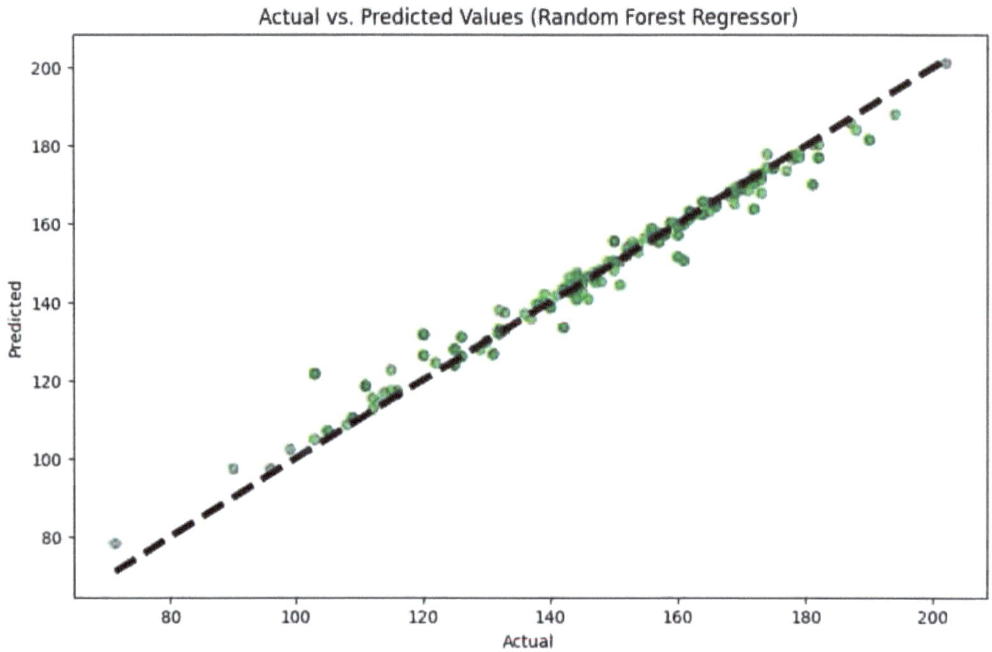

Fig. (4). Random forest regressor result.

The graph in Fig. (**5**) showcases a comparison between the actual 'thalach' values and those predicted by the Gradient Boosting Regressor, with blue dots indicating the predictions and a dashed black line representing the line of perfect prediction. The concentration of blue dots around the dashed line suggests that the Gradient Boosting Regressor has a high predictive accuracy. The distribution of points implies that the model captures the underlying trend effectively, although there are some instances of over- or underestimation, particularly for higher values. The Gradient Boosting Regressor exhibits a strong ability to predict the 'thalach' value, as evidenced by the close fit to the line of perfect prediction. The slight deviations in higher values suggest that there is a room for further tuning, but overall, the model appears to be a potent tool for this predictive task.

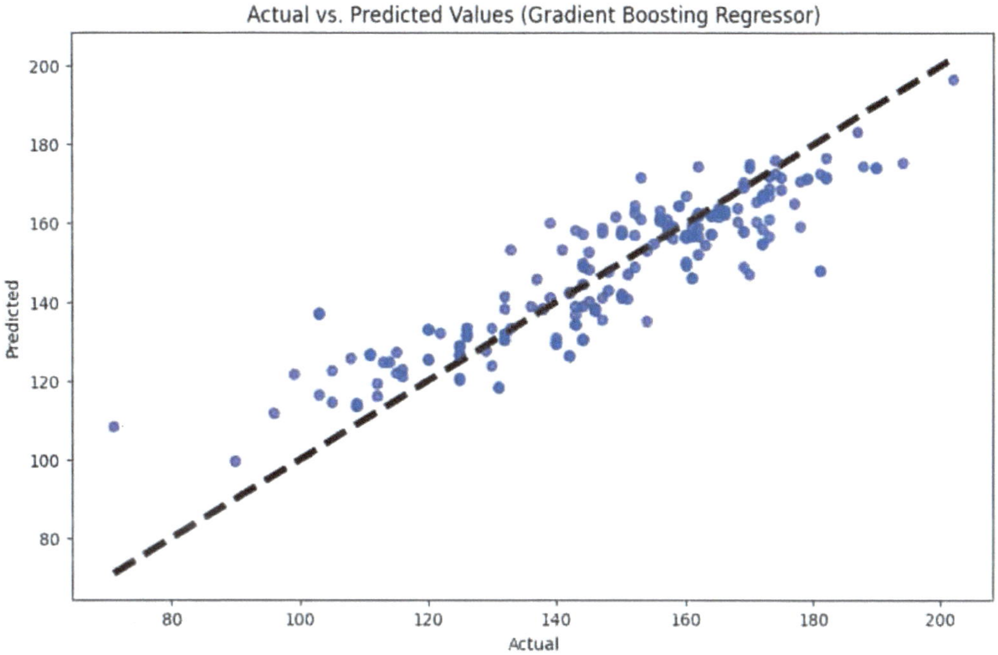

Fig. (5). Gradient boosting regressor result.

Table **1** shows the evaluation of the performance of different machine learning methods. The models were evaluated based on their MSE, MAE, and R^2 metrics for the dataset. The Random Forest Regressor showed significantly lower MSE and MAE values and higher R^2 values for the dataset, indicating superior performance in predicting the heart rate. For the tested dataset, the Random Forest Regressor is the best model, given its highest R^2 score and lowest error metrics. Based on the comparative analysis, the following recommendations are made for model implementation: The Random Forest Regressor should be used for the dataset, as it provides the most accurate and reliable predictions.

Table 1. Evaluation of the performance of different models for the tested dataset.

Model	MSE	MAE	R^2
LinearRegression	283.690883	13.259960	0.462960
Random Forest Regressor	18.895370	2.681845	0.964230
Gradient Boosting Regressor	115.191848	8.174055	0.781937

CONCLUSION

The investigation into using machine learning to predict the maximum heart rate achievable by individuals underscores the transformative potential of ML in the healthcare domain. The Random Forest Regressor emerged as the most effective model for the dataset, demonstrating the highest accuracy and reliability. The study highlighted key challenges, including handling imbalanced datasets and ensuring model interpretability, which is pivotal for clinical applicability. Future work could expand on integrating deeper learning models and more diverse datasets, including longitudinal data, to enhance predictive performance further. Other machine learning models with optimization techniques can also be adapted for the current problem. Ultimately, this chapter lays the groundwork for leveraging machine learning to pioneer advancements in cardiovascular health monitoring and preventive care, marking a step forward in personalized and predictive healthcare.

REFERENCES

[1] Alhussan AA, Abdelhamid AA, Towfek SK, *et al.* Classification of diabetes using feature selection and hybrid al-biruni earth radius and dipper throated optimization. Diagnostics (Basel) 2023; 13(12): 2038.
[http://dx.doi.org/10.3390/diagnostics13122038] [PMID: 37370932]

[2] Alharbi AH, Towfek SK, Abdelhamid AA, *et al.* Diagnosis of monkeypox disease using transfer learning and binary advanced dipper throated optimization algorithm. Biomimetics (Basel) 2023; 8(3): 313.
[http://dx.doi.org/10.3390/biomimetics8030313] [PMID: 37504202]

[3] Eid MM, El-Kenawy ESM, Khodadadi N, *et al.* Meta-heuristic optimization of LSTM-based deep network for boosting the prediction of monkeypox cases. Mathematics 2022; 10(20): 3845.
[http://dx.doi.org/10.3390/math10203845]

[4] Atteia G, Abdel Samee N, El-Kenawy ESM, Ibrahim A. CNN-hyperparameter optimization for diabetic maculopathy diagnosis in optical coherence tomography and fundus retinography. Mathematics 2022; 10(18): 3274.
[http://dx.doi.org/10.3390/math10183274]

[5] El-kenawy ESM, Mirjalili S, Khodadadi N, *et al.* Feature selection in wind speed forecasting systems based on meta-heuristic optimization. PLoS One 2023; 18(2): e0278491.
[http://dx.doi.org/10.1371/journal.pone.0278491] [PMID: 36749744]

[6] Draper, N. R., & Smith, H. (1998). Applied Regression Analysis. John Wiley & Sons. This book is a comprehensive resource on regression analysis, providing theoretical foundations and practical applications.
[http://dx.doi.org/10.1002/9781118625590]

[7] Breiman L. Random Forests. Mach Learn 2001; 45(1): 5-32. [This seminal paper introduces the Random Forest algorithm, detailing its operation and applications.].
[http://dx.doi.org/10.1023/A:1010933404324]

[8] Friedman JH. Greedy function approximation: A gradient boosting machine. Ann Stat 2001; 29(5): 1189-232. [This paper describes the theory and practical implementation of Gradient Boosting Machines, a cornerstone in understanding the algorithm.].
[http://dx.doi.org/10.1214/aos/1013203451]

[9] Khafaga DS, Ibrahim A, El-Kenawy ESM, *et al.* An al-biruni earth radius optimization-based deep convolutional neural network for classifying monkeypox disease. Diagnostics (Basel) 2022; 12(11): 2892.
[http://dx.doi.org/10.3390/diagnostics12112892] [PMID: 36428952]

[10] Shams MY, Elshewey AM, El-kenawy ESM, Ibrahim A, Talaat FM, Tarek Z. Water quality prediction using machine learning models based on grid search method. Multimedia Tools Appl 2023; 83(12): 35307-34.
[http://dx.doi.org/10.1007/s11042-023-16737-4]

[11] El-Kenawy EM, Zerouali B, Bailek N, *et al.* Improved weighted ensemble learning for predicting the daily reference evapotranspiration under the semi-arid climate conditions. Environ Sci Pollut Res Int 2022; 29(54): 81279-99.
[http://dx.doi.org/10.1007/s11356-022-21410-8] [PMID: 35731435]

[12] El-Sayed M. El-kenawy, Abdelaziz A. Abdelhamid, Abdelhameed Ibrahim, Seyedali Mirjalili, Nima Khodadad, Mona A. Al duailij, Amel Ali Alhussan, Doaa Sami Khafaga, Al-Biruni Earth Radius (BER) Metaheuristic Search Optimization Algorithm. Comput Syst Sci Eng 2023; 45(2): 1917-34.
[http://dx.doi.org/10.32604/csse.2023.032497]

[13] Pedregosa F, Varoquaux G, Gramfort A, *et al.* Scikit-learn: Machine Learning in python. J Mach Learn Res 2011; 12: 2825-30.

[14] Abbasi, F. Heart Diseases prediction with streamlit, 2022. Available from: https://www.kaggle.com/datasets/faresabbasai2022/heart-diseases-prediction-with-streamlit/data

CHAPTER 8

Machine Learning Models for Analyzing Diabetes Datasets to Predict Disease Progression and Patient Outcomes

Yaqoob Alhasan[1] and **Abdelhameed Ibrahim**[1,*]

[1] *Faculty of Engineering, Design and Information & Communications Technology (EDICT), School of ICT, Bahrain Polytechnic, PO Box 33349, Isa Town, Bahrain*

Abstract: Machine learning is central in analyzing numerical diabetes datasets to predict disease progression and patient outcomes. The primary objective is to develop a model that accurately forecasts the patient's future health status based on historical and current medical data. Predictive analytics is essential for early intervention and personalized patient care. The chapter focuses on the pressing healthcare challenge of diabetes, a pervasive condition characterized by significant complexity and requiring precise diagnostic measures. Recognizing the ample data available on diabetes and the severe complications associated with the disease, there is an imperative demand for enhancing the accuracy of its diagnosis. The dataset utilized in this chapter was meticulously compiled from patient records within the Iraqi healthcare system, specifically sourced from the Medical City Hospital's laboratory and the Specialized Center for Endocrinology and Diabetes at Al-Kindy Teaching Hospital. To advance the diagnosis and predictive modeling of diabetes, a comprehensive dataset was curated, drawing from a wide range of medical and laboratory analysis records. This dataset was pivotal in fostering a deeper understanding of the multifactorial nature of diabetes within Iraqi society. Support Vector Regression (SVR), Random Forest Regressor, and K-Nearest Neighbors Regressor (KNN) were applied to the tested dataset. In the experimental results, the SVR model showed the most significant improvement post-optimization, with substantial decreases in Mean Squared Error (MSE), Root Mean Squared Error (RMSE), and Mean Absolute Error (MAE), and a notable increase in R^2, indicating a substantial enhancement in both the model's accuracy and its explanatory power.

Keywords: Diabetes, K-nearest neighbors regressor, Machine learning, Random forest regressor, Support vector regression.

[*] **Corresponding author Abdelhameed Ibrahim:** Faculty of Engineering, Design and Information & Communications Technology (EDICT), School of ICT, Bahrain Polytechnic, PO Box 33349, Isa Town, Bahrain;
E-mail: abdelhameed.fawzy@polytechnic.bh

Neeraj Gupta, Abdelhameed Ibrahim, Bhavesh Vyas & Shobhna Jeet (Eds.)

INTRODUCTION

The prevalence of diabetes worldwide is a growing health concern, leading to an increased need for predictive models that can accurately forecast diabetes progression and complications based on patient data [1]. Machine learning models can be crucial in predicting such outcomes, which can be instrumental in preventive healthcare and resource optimization. However, the challenge lies in accurately modeling the progression of diabetes using clinical data, which is often heterogeneous and contains numerous potential predictors [2, 3]. The primary objective of this chapter is to process two distinct numerical datasets related to diabetes by cleaning data, which includes removing irrelevant features and handling missing values to create a robust dataset for model training.

Machine learning can be essential in discovering medical risk factors using data-driven methods [4, 5]. Three different machine learning regression models are selected to be applied to predict various diabetes-related outcomes: Support Vector Regression (SVR), Random Forest Regressor, and K-Nearest Neighbors Regressor (KNN) [6]. The model training is performed using the preprocessed dataset, and the initial performance is evaluated to establish a baseline for comparison. To assess the final models' performance on a separate test subset and generate comprehensive reports that include prediction error and original versus prediction analysis, insights are provided into each model's accuracy and precision.

The software libraries and packages involved in the execution of the machine learning project focused on diabetes dataset analysis and predictive modeling. The pandas (pd) package is used for data manipulation and analysis. It is used for reading, writing, and processing data from various file formats, as well as handling missing data. The NumPy (np) package is used for numerical computing with Python, which supports multi-dimensional arrays and provides mathematical functions to operate on array elements. The Matplotlib.pyplot (plt) is applied to the Python 2D plotting library. It includes creating static, interactive, and animated visualizations in Python. It is helpful for plotting graphs, histograms, and scatterplots.

The preprocessing and data cleaning process for completing missing values, including replacing these values encoded as np.nan using the mean, median, or most frequent value along each column, is performed based on Scikit-learn's Impute.SimpleImputer package. The standardization of the dataset for scaling features to center around zero with a standard deviation of one, essential for many machine learning algorithms, is applied using Scikit-learn's Preprocessing. StandardScaler package. Scaling each feature to a given range is performed by

Scikit-learn's Preprocessing.MinMaxScaler, which includes scaling a feature to a chosen range, often between zero and one. The last preprocessing step for encoding labels with values between 0 and n classes-1, including converting categorical text data into a model-understandable numerical format, is performed by Scikit-learn's Preprocessing.LabelEncoder.

The machine learning algorithms of the Scikit-Learn library include Scikit-learn's SVM.SVR, Scikit-learn's Ensemble.RandomForestRegressor, and Scikit-learn's Neighbors.KNeighborsRegressor. The training and evaluation of the machine learning model are performed using Scikit-learn's Model Selection. train_test_split and Scikit-learn's Metrics packages. Splitting arrays or matrices into random trains and test subsets, including splitting the dataset into training and testing sets for model validation, is a fundamental step in machine learning. The metrics for measuring model performance include mean_squared_error and mean_absolute_error, which evaluate the performance of the models.

Support Vector Regression (SVR) is applied in the context of regression problems. Random Forest Regressor and K-Nearest Neighbors Regressor (KNN) are also applied to the tested dataset. The KNN algorithm searches for 'k' nearest instances in the training dataset and averages their values to make a prediction. In the experimental results for the dataset, the SVR model shows the most significant improvement post-optimization, with substantial decreases in Mean Squared Error (MSE), Root Mean Squared Error (RMSE), and Mean Absolute Error (MAE), and a notable increase in R^2, indicating a substantial enhancement in both the model's accuracy and its explanatory power. The KNN model shows marginal improvements in MSE, RMSE, and MAE and a slight increase in R^2. The improvement is positive but not as pronounced as SVR. The Random Forest Regressor performed worse post-optimization, with increases in MSE, RMSE, and MAE and a decrease in R^2. This indicates that the optimization may not have been effective, or the model may have overfit the training data and thus performed poorly on the test set. After parameter optimization, the SVR model outperforms the other two models on the second dataset.

METHODOLOGY

Dataset and Evaluation Metrics

For the regression task, a numerical-related application and topic dataset (Diabetes Predictions) are used [7]. For implementation, the Python programming language is applied using Pandas, NumPy, Scikit-learn packages for machine learning algorithms, and Matplotlib for visualization. For the dataset preprocessing, the process includes:

- Dropping all categorical columns and keeping the numerical ones.
- Handling the Missing Values (Null Values) by filling the missing rows with the mean method.
- Setting the criteria to select the most relevant column between the tested dataset and choosing it to be the targeted column.

The metrics of MSE, RMSE, MAE, MBE, and R-squared value are used to further evaluate the model fit [8].

Model Selection

For the machine learning models, three regression models (k-Nearest Neighbors Regressor, Random Forest Regressor, Support Vector Regressor) are selected to be applied to the tested dataset.

Support Vector Regression (SVR)

The SVR is applied in the context of regression problems. It works primarily by focusing on minimizing error within a certain margin. SVR is used for regression tasks, mainly when dealing with small datasets. SVR is chosen for its effectiveness and its ability to model complex, non-linear relationships in the data [9, 10]. The parameters of Kernel, Epsilon, C, and Gamma are adjusted to the SVR model as follows.

- Kernel: rbf (Radial Basis Function) for a non-linear transformation of the input space.
- Epsilon: 0.1, determining the margin of tolerance where no penalty is given to errors.
- C: 1.5, setting the trade-off between the smoothness of the regression function.
- Gamma: 0.05, defining the influence of a single training example.

Random Forest Regressor

Random Forest is an ensemble learning method for regression that operates based on decision trees. The choice of an ensemble method, specifically Random Forest, is due to its ability to reduce overfitting without substantially increasing error due to bias, as well as its performance in various benchmark studies [11, 12]. The parameters are adjusted as follows.

- n_estimators: Optimal number determined by Grey Wolf Optimizer (GWO), indicating the number of trees in the forest.

- max_depth: Optimal depth of the tree, ensuring sufficient complexity to capture data patterns without overfitting.
- min_samples_split and min_samples_leaf.

K-Nearest Neighbors Regressor (KNN)

KNN operates on the principle that similar data points can be predicted by their proximity to each other. This algorithm searches for 'k' nearest instances in the training dataset and averages their values to make a prediction. KNN was selected for its simplicity and non-parametric nature, making it suitable for regression problems where the relationship between variables is poorly understood [13, 14]. KNN demonstrated moderate performance with slightly higher errors compared to other models. However, its value lies in the interpretability and straightforward application without the need for extensive parameter tuning. The parameters are as follows.

- n_neighbors: 5, to determine the number of neighbors to consider.
- Weights: distance, giving preference to nearer neighbors.
- Algorithm: kd_tree, an efficient method for nearest neighbors?(tm) search.

EVALUATE THE PERFORMANCE OF MODELS

In this section, the results of the evaluation of the machine learning model?(tm)s performance are presented and discussed based on the tested dataset in a model's [7].

SVR (Support Vector Regression) for Tested Dataset

Table **1** presents the output values based on changing the regularization parameter (C) from 1.0 to 1.5. Fig. (**1**) shows the tested dataset for the regularization parameter C. Fig. (**2**) shows the tested dataset prediction by SVR for post-optimization of the regularization parameter C.

Table 1. SVR results by changing the regularization parameter (C) from 1.0 to 1.5

PRE-OPTIMIZATION (C=1.0):		POST-OPTIMIZATION (C=1.5):	
MSE	0.006818149	MSE	0.006888193
RMSE	0.082572085	RMSE	0.082995136
MAE	0.058681506	MAE	0.059356119
MBE	-0.041436312	MBE	-0.042381775
R^2	0.035526234	R^2	0.03632623

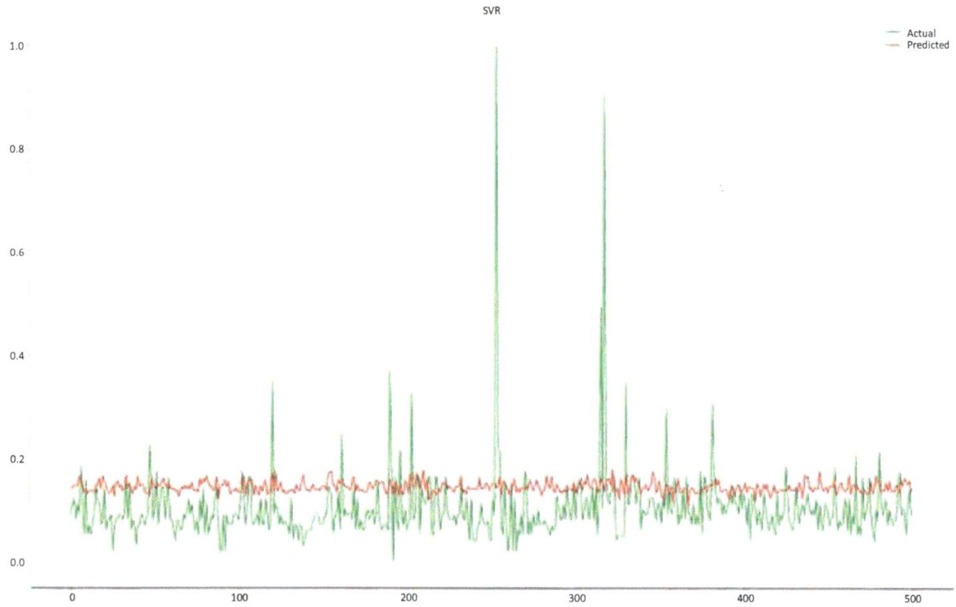

Fig. (1). Tested dataset prediction by SVR for pre-optimization case.

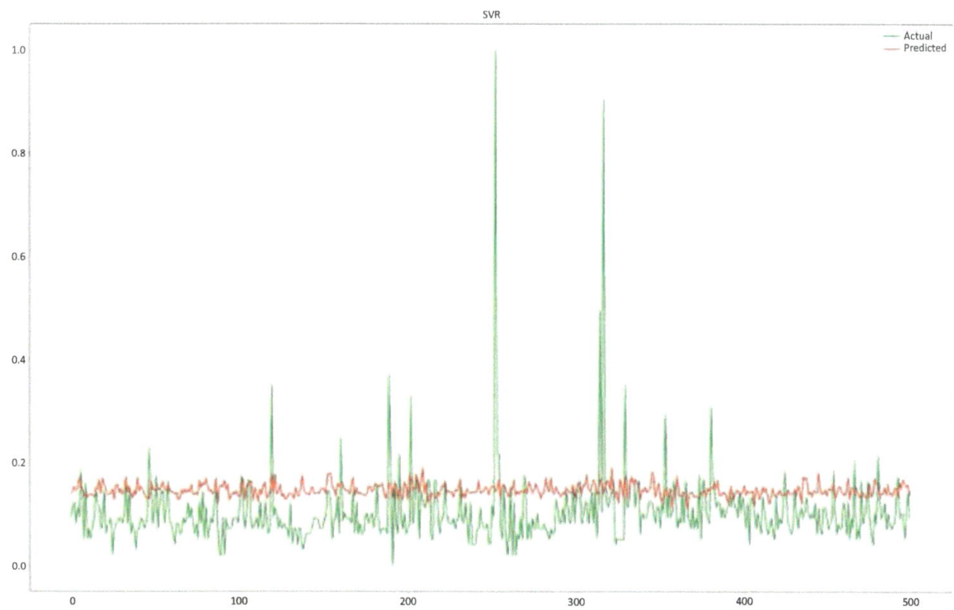

Fig. (2). Tested dataset prediction by SVR for post-optimization case.

The results of the Support Vector Regression (SVR) model before and after optimization can be explained as follows. The MSE value for the pre-optimization case was 0.006818149, and for the post-optimization case, it was 0.006888193, suggesting that it slightly increased after increasing C from 1.0 to 1.5. This suggests that the model with a higher C value is slightly less accurate on the training data. The RMSE value for pre-optimization was 0.082572085, and for post-optimization, it was 0.082995136. The increase in RMSE indicates that the data points are, on average, further away from the regression line after optimization. The MAE value of pre-optimization was 0.058681506, and it was 0.059356119 for post-optimization. The slight increase in MAE post-optimization suggests that the average error in prediction increased with a higher C value. A negative value indicates an overall underprediction. The increase in the magnitude of the negative MBE value indicates that increasing C led to a slight increase in the bias of under-prediction. A slight increase in R^2 suggests a minimal improvement in the model's explanatory power after optimization.

After increasing the regularization parameter C from 1.0 to 1.5, the model shows a slight deterioration in prediction accuracy (as shown by MSE and RMSE) and an increase in the average error (MAE). However, the model has a marginally increased R^2 value, suggesting a negligible improvement in how well the future samples are likely to be predicted by the model. It is worth noting that all changes are quite small, so the practical significance of increasing C in this context may be limited. This could mean that the model is relatively stable with respect to changes in C, or it could indicate that other parameters or features substantially impact model performance.

Random Forest Regressor

This section presents the Random Forest Regressor optimized with the Grey Wolf Optimizer (GWO) and its pre- and post-optimization values. Table **2** presents the output results of Random Forest before and after optimization by the Grey Wolf Optimizer. Fig. (**3**) shows the dataset by Random Forest Regressor pre-optimization, and Fig. (**4**) presents the dataset by Random Forest Regressor post-optimization.

Table 2. Random Forest results before and after optimization by Grey Wolf Optimizer

PRE-OPTIMIZATION:		POST-OPTIMIZATION:	
MSE	0.006730738	**MSE**	0.005547105
RMSE	0.082041075	**RMSE**	0.074478888
MAE	0.042213055	**MAE**	0.03727988
MBE	-0.009276435	**MBE**	-0.001809684
R^2	0.007872526	R^2	0.012067864

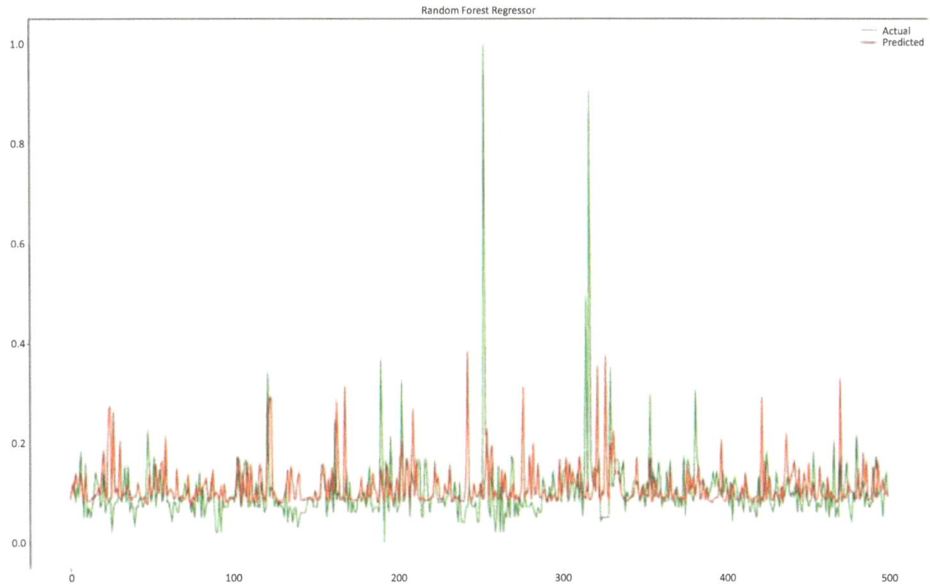

Fig. (3). Tested dataset by Random Forest Regressor pre-optimization.

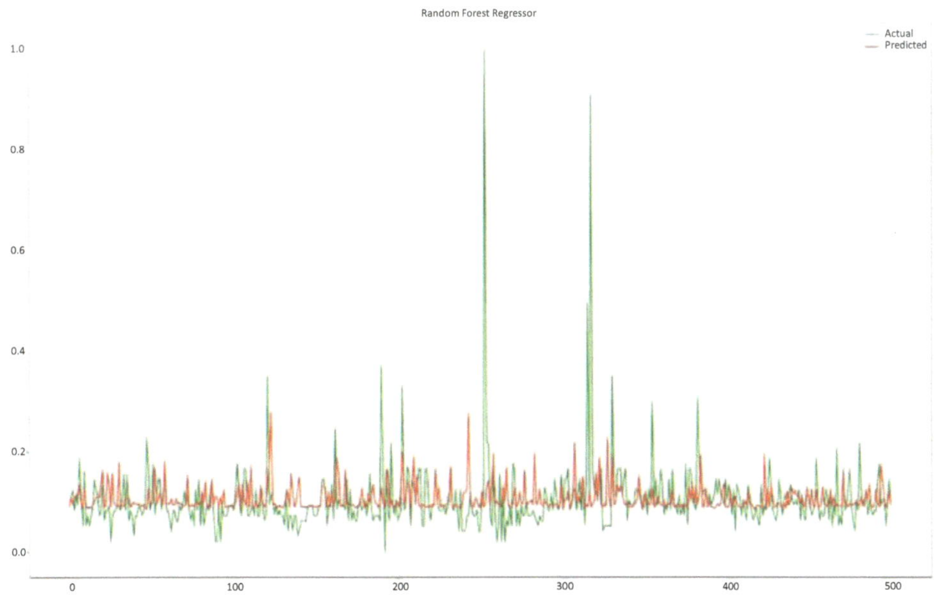

Fig. (4). Tested dataset by Random Forest Regressor post-optimization.

MSE decreased after optimization, indicating that the differences between the observed and predicted values are lower. This suggests an improvement in the model's predictive accuracy. It shows a decrease as well. Lower RMSE values indicate a better fit as the residuals (prediction errors) are smaller, meaning the optimized model's predictions are closer to the actual values. The decrease in MAE shows that the mean absolute value of the errors has reduced. The optimization has led to predictions that are, on average, more accurate, and the deviation from actual values is less. MBE is closer to zero after optimization, which indicates a reduction in systematic bias. The negative sign indicates under-prediction, but the magnitude of under-prediction is less post-optimization, suggesting that the model is now more balanced in its predictions. An increase in the R^2 value post-optimization is noticeable.

GWO seems to have significantly improved the performance of the Random Forest Regressor across all metrics. The post-optimization model is more accurate (lower MSE and MAE), has a better fit (lower RMSE), is less biased (MBE closer to zero), and is generally more effective at predicting the variance in the dataset (higher R^2). This suggests that the optimization has successfully found hyperparameter settings that produce a more accurate and reliable model.

KNN (K-Nearest Neighbors Regressor)

This section presents the KNN Regressor pre-optimization and post-optimization values. Table **3** shows the output results of KNN before and after optimization by adding distance-based weighting and the KD tree algorithm for Nearest Neighbor Search. Fig. (**5**) shows the dataset by KNN Regressor pre-optimization, and Fig. (**6**) presents the dataset by KNN Regressor post-optimization.

Table 3. KNN results before and after optimization

PRE-OPTIMIZATION:		POST OPTIMIZATION:	
MSE	0.00577013	**MSE**	0.005730058
RMSE	0.07596137	**RMSE**	0.075697147
MAE	0.039094433	**MAE**	0.038723803
MBE	0.003869691	**MBE**	0.004343876
R^2	0.013731135	**R^2**	0.014974034

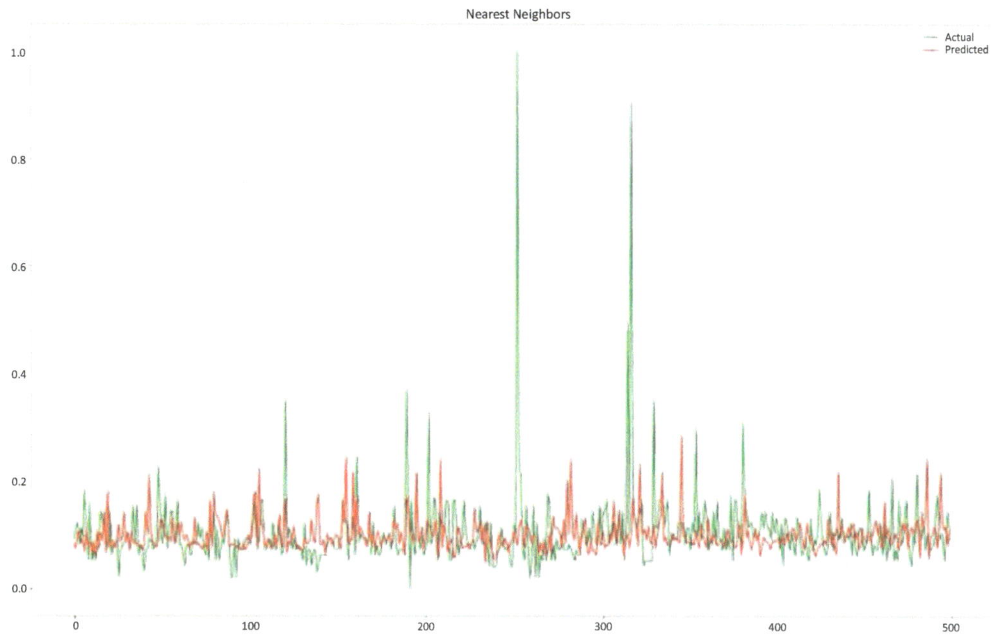

Fig. (5). Tested dataset by the KNN Regressor pre-optimization.

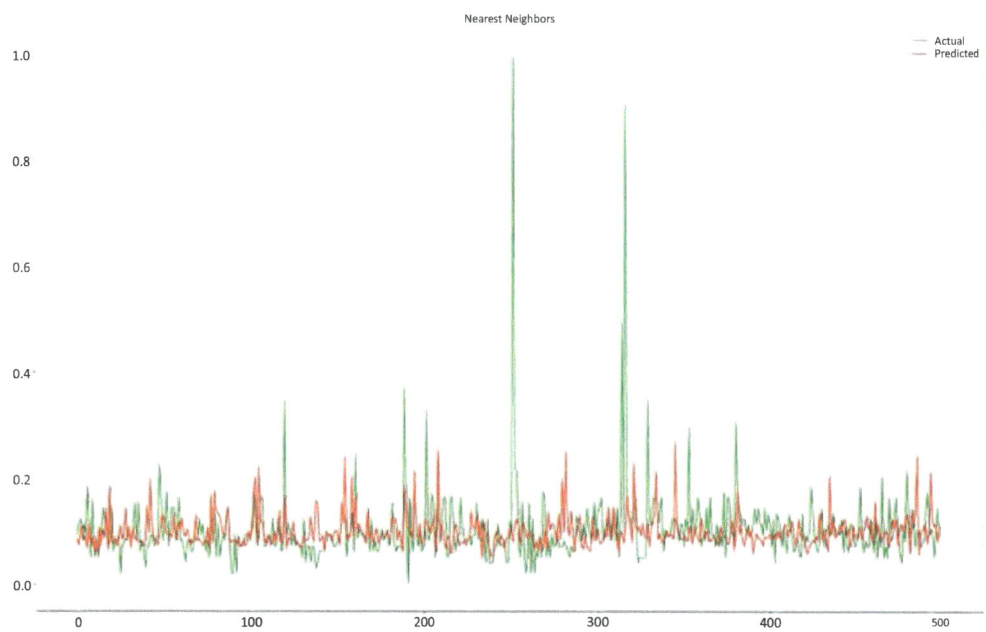

Fig. (6). Tested dataset by KNN Regressor post-optimization.

The MSE slightly decreased after optimization, which means that the value has reduced, indicating a slight improvement in the precision of the model's predictions. The RMSE decreased post-optimization, suggesting that the standard deviation of the residuals has become smaller. Hence, the model's predictions are more concentrated around the actual values. The MAE marginally decreased, indicating that, on average, the absolute errors between the predicted and actual values are slightly lower. This suggests a modest improvement in the model's accuracy. MBE increased in magnitude, suggesting a slight increase in the systematic bias in the model post-optimization, with the model tending to slightly over-predict the target values more than before. The R^2 value increased, which indicates that the model is now slightly better at explaining the variance in the dataset. The proportion of the total variation of outcomes explained by the model improved, which is a positive sign.

After optimization, which involved adding distance-based weighting and using the KD tree algorithm for nearest neighbor search, the KNN model showed marginal improvements in MSE, RMSE, and MAE, suggesting better accuracy and a tighter fit to the data. However, the increase in MBE suggests that the model's predictions have more systematic overestimation than before. The increase in R^2, while still very small, implies that the model's ability to explain the variability of the response variable improved slightly. Overall, the changes are minimal, suggesting that the KNN model's performance is relatively stable to these parameter changes for this dataset.

DISCUSSION

The Random Forest Regressor showed improvements across all metrics, indicating that it performed better and had the most substantial improvement overall after optimization. The KNN model showed slight improvements across all metrics, but to a lesser extent than the Random Forest. The SVR model, while slightly improving R^2, performed worse in terms of MSE, RMSE, and MAE, suggesting that the parameter change (regularization parameter C) did not positively impact the model performance for this dataset. The Random Forest Regressor model performed the best on the dataset and exhibited the most significant improvement after optimization with the Grey Wolf Optimizer. Its lower errors and higher R^2 value post-optimization suggest that it is the most suitable model for this specific dataset.

CONCLUSION

Machine learning plays a central role in analyzing numerical diabetes datasets to predict disease progression and patient outcomes. The primary objective is to develop a model that accurately forecasts the patient's future health status based on historical and current medical data. This kind of predictive analytics is essential for early intervention and personalized patient care. The models were trained on numerical diabetes datasets that include various physiological and medical test variables. SVR, Random Forest, and KNN are the three regression models chosen for implementation in this project. These models were trained to identify and learn patterns within the dataset. The optimization process for each model involved tuning hyperparameters, specifically the regularization parameter C in the SVR model, and optimizing the Random Forest model with the GWO. For the KNN model, distance weighting and algorithm choice for nearest neighbors were optimized.

A range of metrics was used in this chapter to evaluate and compare model performance, pre- and post-optimization. The measures of MSE, RMSE, MAE, MBE, and R^2 were used to gain a better understanding of how well the model's predictions align with the actual outcomes.

REFERENCES

[1] Ellulu MS, Samouda H. Clinical and biological risk factors associated with inflammation in patients with type 2 diabetes mellitus. BMC Endocr Disord 2022; 22(1): 16.
[http://dx.doi.org/10.1186/s12902-021-00925-0] [PMID: 34991564]

[2] Alhussan AA, Abdelhamid AA, Towfek SK, *et al.* Classification of diabetes using feature selection and hybrid al-biruni earth radius and dipper throated optimization. Diagnostics (Basel) 2023; 13(12): 2038.
[http://dx.doi.org/10.3390/diagnostics13122038] [PMID: 37370932]

[3] Atteia G, Abdel Samee N, El-Kenawy ESM, Ibrahim A. CNN-hyperparameter optimization for diabetic maculopathy diagnosis in optical coherence tomography and fundus retinography. Mathematics 2022; 10(18): 3274.
[http://dx.doi.org/10.3390/math10183274]

[4] Alharbi AH, Towfek SK, Abdelhamid AA, *et al.* Diagnosis of monkeypox disease using transfer learning and binary advanced dipper throated optimization algorithm. Biomimetics (Basel) 2023; 8(3): 313.
[http://dx.doi.org/10.3390/biomimetics8030313] [PMID: 37504202]

[5] Eid MM, El-Kenawy ESM, Khodadadi N, *et al.* Meta-heuristic optimization of LSTM-based deep network for boosting the prediction of monkeypox cases. Mathematics 2022; 10(20): 3845.
[http://dx.doi.org/10.3390/math10203845]

[6] El-kenawy ESM, Mirjalili S, Khodadadi N, *et al.* Feature selection in wind speed forecasting systems based on meta-heuristic optimization. PLoS One 2023; 18(2): e0278491.
[http://dx.doi.org/10.1371/journal.pone.0278491] [PMID: 36749744]

[7] ADiabetes Dataset. (n.d.). Www.kaggle.com. Retrieved April 6, 2024, Available from: https://www.kaggle.com/datasets/aravindpcoder/diabetes-dataset/data

[8] H., Faris., Elshabrawy, Mahmoud., Sameh, Basant., Mohamed, Karim., Mohamed, Ahmed. Optimizing student performance prediction using binary waterwheel plant algorithm for feature selection and machine learning. Journal of Artificial Intelligence and Metaheuristics, vol. , no. , 2024, pp. 19-37.
[http://dx.doi.org/10.54216/JAIM.070102]

[9] Kumar, Manish. , H., Faris. , Elshabrawy, Mahmoud. , Mohamed, Ahmed. Predicting student

outcomes: Evaluating regression techniques in educational data. Journal of Artificial Intelligence and Metaheuristics, vol., no., 2024, pp. 51-62. [http://dx.doi.org/10.54216/JAIM.070205]

[10] H., Faris., Saleh, Ahmed., Elgaml, Abdulrhman., Elsakaan, Ahmed., Mohamed, Ahmed. Exploring predictive models for students' performance in exams: A comparative analysis of regression algorithms. Journal of Artificial Intelligence and Metaheuristics, vol. , no. , 2024, pp. 38-52. [http://dx.doi.org/10.54216/JAIM.070103]

[11] El-Sayed M. El-kenawy, Abdelhameed Ibrahim, Seyedali Mirjalili, Yu-Dong Zhang, Shaima Elnazer, Rokaia M. Zaki, Optimized ensemble algorithm for predicting metamaterial antenna parameters, computers. Materials & Continua 2022; 71(3): 4989-5003. [http://dx.doi.org/10.32604/cmc.2022.023884]

[12] IBM. (n.d.). What is random forest? From IBM: Available from: https://www.ibm.com/topics/random-forest Last visited 1-08-2024

[13] El-Kenawy ESM, Khodadadi N, Mirjalili S, *et al.* Metaheuristic optimization for improving weed detection in wheat images captured by drones. Mathematics 2022; 10(23): 4421. [http://dx.doi.org/10.3390/math10234421]

[14] Shams MY, Elshewey AM, El-kenawy ESM, Ibrahim A, Talaat FM, Tarek Z. Water quality prediction using machine learning models based on grid search method. Multimedia Tools Appl 2023; 83(12): 35307-34. [http://dx.doi.org/10.1007/s11042-023-16737-4]

CHAPTER 9

The Impact of Large Language Models on Healthcare

Urvinder Kaur[1,*], **Neeraj Gupta**[1] and **Harminder Kaur**[2]

[1] *Department of Information Technology, Panipat Institute of Engineering and Technology, Samalka, Haryana, India*

[2] *Sharda University, Greater Noida, India*

Abstract: Healthcare will significantly shift, and LLMs will play a significant role in this industry. Retraining the use of medical databases or generic LLMs to finetune might help develop strategies to improve the usability of LLMs for healthcare. Additionally, multimodal LLMs feature fusion using various data sources, including tabular and visual data, which leads to even greater performance than humans. Even though there are many advantages to using LLMs, it is essential to acknowledge that the content created cannot be solely the responsibility of LLMs. To prevent any potential harm, it is crucial to thoroughly evaluate anything AI generates. Reducing the bar for LLM deployments means that there is more time to focus on improving deployment requirements. To better assist clinical decision-making, efforts should encourage incorporating LLMs in medicine, strengthen human-machine collaboration, and enhance LLM interpretability in clinical contexts. Physicians may optimize the advantages of AI while minimizing possible hazards and improving patient outcomes by utilizing LLMs as an auxiliary tool. Ultimately, the cooperation of administrators, patients, data scientists, doctors, and regulatory agencies will be necessary to integrate LLMs into healthcare effectively.

Keywords: AI, Corpus, Data, Ethical relationship, Healthcare, LLM, ML, Medical specialization, Training.

INTRODUCTION

A person's capacity to express and communicate is known as their language. It starts to form in early childhood and keeps evolving throughout their lifetime [1]. Conversely, machines must have the innate capacity to comprehend and exchange information through human language if outfitted with robust Artificial Intelligence (AI) algorithms. The objective of enabling robots to read, write, and

* **Corresponding author Urvinder Kaur:** Department of Information Technology, Panipat Institute of Engineering and Technology, Samalka, Haryana, India; E-mail: urvinder.it@piet.co.in

Neeraj Gupta, Abdelhameed Ibrahim, Bhavesh Vyas & Shobhna Jeet (Eds.)

converse like humans has long been a scientific problem [2]. Strictly speaking, one of the main strategies for increasing machine language intelligence is Language Modeling (LM). LM generally attempts to forecast the probability of future (or absent) tokens by modeling the generative likelihood of word sequences.

Large Language Models (LLMs) have gained immense interest in the last five years. These models have self-attention capabilities, and they can extract and understand the meaning and relationship between words and phrases in a sentence. These large-scale unsupervised models are trained on an enormous amount of data to enable them to generate coherent and contextually relevant responses. LLMs have found applications in various domains, including healthcare, entertainment, transportation, education, etc.

Large Language Models (LLMs) are set to revolutionize healthcare. They can enhance clinical decision support, automate administrative tasks, and improve patient engagement. LLMs have applications in various medical specialties, offering innovative solutions for diagnostics and patient care. However, integrating LLMs in healthcare faces challenges like data privacy, security concerns, and the need for vast training data. Collaborative efforts between healthcare professionals and data scientists are essential to realize the full potential of LLMs in healthcare. Section 1 of this chapter reviews the background of large language models.

BACKGROUND OF LLMS

Language models are probabilistic models used for various text-based natural language processing tasks. LLMs are the latest form of language models. They combine large data sets, neural networks, and transformers. This section covers the four main phases of development in LM research:

- Statistical Language Models (SLM). The prominent statistical learning methods in the 1990s generated SLMs [3]. The primary objective is to create a word prediction model based on the Markov assumption, for example, using the most recent context to anticipate the following phrase. Bigram and trigram language models are examples of SLMs. These language models extensively improve task performance in Natural Language Processing (NLP) and information retrieval [4, 5]. Nevertheless, high-order language models endure the "curse of dimensionality," making it challenging to predict exponential transition probabilities.
- Neural Language Models (NLM). Using neural networks, such as recurrent neural networks and multi-layer perceptrons, NLMs [6] define the probability of

word sequences. A study [7] significantly contributed to this by creating and expanding the concept of learning efficient features for text input conditioned on the aggregated context information and presenting the idea of distributed representation of words. Generic neural network techniques expanded the concept of learning efficient features for text input to create a comprehensive solution for a range of NLP applications. Moreover, Word2Vec is a technique that builds a more straightforward, shallow neural network to learn distributed word representations. It was introduced and quickly gained popularity in various natural language processing applications. This research has significantly influenced the area of NLP by introducing the representation learning application of language models.

- Pre-trained Language Models (PLM). An early technique called ELMo [8] included pre-training a bidirectional long short-term memory network and optimizing it according to specific downstream tasks. This allowed for learning fixed word representations rather than context-aware word representations. These pre-trained context-aware word representations have significantly raised the bar for Natural Language Processing (NLP) tasks and are instrumental as all-purpose semantic features. This work has motivated numerous follow-up studies and established the paradigm for “pretraining and finetuning” learning. Much work on PLMs has been created after this framework, presenting distinct designs such as GPT-2 [9]. According to this paradigm, the PLM must frequently adjust to various requirements and conditions.
- Large Language Models (LLM). Researchers discover that improving model capability frequently results from scaling PLM [10]. Many experiments have trained ever-larger PLMs to investigate the performance limit. These larger PLMs behave differently from smaller PLMs and demonstrate unexpected capabilities in resolving several challenging tasks despite scaling primarily done in model size. These huge-sized PLMs, garnering more and more interest from researchers, are referred to by the academic community as “Large Language Models (LLM).” One outstanding use of LLMs is ChatGPT2, which transforms the GPT series LLMs into dialogue and offers incredible human communication capabilities. Thus, one type of Artificial Intelligence (AI) produced by training neural networks on massive amounts of textual data is Large Language Models (LLMs). Source code and other innovative human-like outputs may be made quickly by LLMs.

KEY TECHNIQUES FOR LLM

The evolution of LLMs into broad and competent learners has been a long journey. LLM's success can be attributed to various crucial strategies, as discussed below:

- **Scaling:** Scaling refers to the model's quality depending on the training data volume and computation resources. Transformer language models exhibit a scaling effect; more training computation and larger model/data volumes often result in higher model capacities [11]. GPT-3 and PaLM, two exemplary models, were used to investigate the scaling limitations. Their respective sizes were increased to 175B and 540B. Scaling rules can be utilized alongside the compute budget, which is often limited, to distribute the computing resources more efficiently. For example, by expanding the data set while keeping the same computing budget, Chinchilla (with more training tokens) performs better than Gopher (with a bigger model size). Furthermore, as the quality of the pretraining data is a significant factor in the model's ability, data should be scaled carefully after cleaning.
- **Training:** Training a proficient LLM is challenging because of the large model size. Distributed training methods are needed to learn the network parameters of LLMs, which sometimes involve multiple parallel procedures. DeepSpeed and Megatron-LM are two examples of optimization frameworks made available to allow distributed training and make it easier to install and apply parallel algorithms. Optimization strategies such as restarting to overcome a training loss spike and using mixed precision training are essential for training stability and model performance. More recently, GPT-4 suggests creating specialized frameworks and optimization techniques that may accurately forecast large-scale model performance using much smaller models [12].
- **Ability eliciting:** Following extensive pretraining on large-scale datasets, LLMs can perform various tasks. These skills may not always be evident when LLMs carry out particular activities. Creating appropriate task instructions or particular in-context learning procedures is helpful as a technical approach to elicit such talents. By incorporating intermediate reasoning processes, chain-of-thought prompting, for example, has been demonstrated to be effective in solving complex reasoning tasks. Moreover, task descriptions written in plain language may be used for LLM instruction tailoring, increasing the generalizability of LLMs on functions.
- **Alignment tuning:** LLMs can extract features from pretraining corpora with high-quality and low-quality data. They may produce damaging, discriminatory, or even hazardous information for human consumption. LLMs must align with human values, such as being kind, truthful, and innocent. To this end, InstructGPT uses reinforcement learning with human input to build an efficient tuning strategy that makes LLMs obey the desired instructions. Using intricately planned labeling techniques, it integrates humans into the training loop. ChatGPT uses a methodology akin to InstructGPT, generating replies, such as refusing to respond to offensive inquiries [13].

- **Tools manipulation**. Essentially, large-scale plain text corpora are used to train language models as text generators. This makes them less effective at tasks not best suited to them, such as numerical calculation. Furthermore, their capabilities are restricted to the pretraining data; for example, they cannot catch current information. One newly suggested method to address these problems is using outside technologies to compensate for LLMs' shortcomings [14]. For instance, LLMs can use search engines to find unfamiliar information and the calculator to perform precise calculations. A system like this can significantly increase the range of capabilities available to LLMs.

PREPARING LLM'S

The foundation of an LLM's talents is established by pretraining. LLMs can learn the fundamentals of language creation and interpretation by pre-training on large-scale corpora [15]. To achieve formidable skills in this process, the size and caliber of the pretraining corpus are crucial. Furthermore, well-designed model architectures, acceleration strategies, and optimization methodologies are necessary for LLM pretraining to be successful. Fig. (**1**) illustrates a typical workflow for preparing the pretraining data for LLMs. This section covers data sources, preprocessing techniques, and a crucial examination of how pretraining data impacts LLM performance.

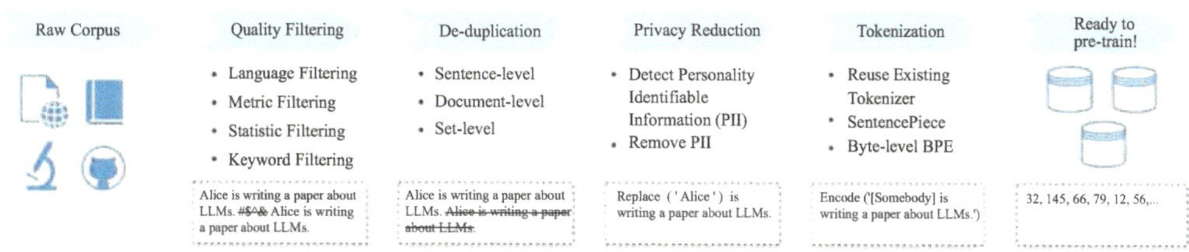

Fig. (1). A typical data preprocessing pipeline for pre-training large language models [16].

Data Source

To create a competent LLM, it is essential to gather a substantial natural language corpus from several sources of information. Current LLMs mostly use a variety of publicly available text datasets as their pretraining corpus. Depending upon the type of application, the data sources for training can be categorized as General Text Data and Specialized Text Data.

General Text Data: General data is vast, varied, and readily available; most LLMs use it to improve their language modeling and generalization skills [17]. Most LLMs use general-purpose pretraining data, which includes rich text sources on various subjects, such as webpages, books, and conversational text.

- **Webpages:** The Internet has made various kinds of data available, which helps LLMs improve their generalization skills and acquire a wide range of linguistic information. A significant quantity of data can be retrieved from the Internet. The crawled online data often contains low-quality text, like spam mail, and high-quality text, like Wikipedia. To improve the quality of data filtering and processing of inputs is of prime importance.
- **Conversation text:** Conversation data can improve LLMs' performance and conversational competency on various question-answering tasks [18]. Scholars may gather conversation data from online social media platforms or use subsets of public discussion corpora [19]. Online conversational data frequently comprises talks between several participants; therefore, turning a conversation into a tree structure, in which each utterance is linked to its response, is an efficient approach to handling the data. This process involves dividing the multi-party conversation tree into smaller discussions, which can be included in the pretraining corpus.
- **Books:** Books offer a significant supply of formal, lengthy texts compared to other corpora, which may help LLMs acquire language skills, simulate long-term reliance, and produce narrative and cohesive works. The author of a study [20] gathered open-source book data from various sources to create an 825 GiB dataset, Pile, to train LLM.

Specialized Text Data: Using three significant categories of specialized datasets can help LLMs do better on specialized tasks.

- **Multilingual text:** A multilingual corpus, in addition to content written in the target language, helps improve multilingual comprehension and linguistic production skills. For example, FLM combines Chinese and English corpora in about equal amounts [21]. These models outperform state-of-the-art models optimized on the corpus in the target language(s) and show outstanding performance in multilingual tasks.
- **Scientific text:** Scientific publications have increased, reflecting human knowledge discovery. Including a scientific corpus for model pretraining helps improve LLMs' comprehension of scientific information. LLMs are adept at scientific and reasoning tasks due to their extensive training in scientific text. Current efforts to build the scientific corpus primarily gather arXiv articles, textbooks, math webpages, and other relevant scientific materials. Because scientific data are complicated, special tokenization and preprocessing approaches are typically needed to unify these disparate data formats into a form that language models can interpret [22].
- **Code:** The research community has extensively examined program synthesis, particularly the application of PLMs trained on code. However, these PLMs

(such as GPT-J) still struggle to produce precise and high-quality programs. According to recent research, training LLMs on a large code corpus can significantly raise the caliber of synthesized programs. The produced programs can solve competitive programming problems and pass expert-designed unit-test cases. Stack Exchange and other programming question-answering forums are the initial sources. The second source is publicly accessible software repositories like GitHub, where code information is gathered, including comments and docstrings.

According to recent research, learning to write code may also be a source of advanced thinking skills, such as the capacity to follow a thought chain. Moreover, encoding reasoning problems into code might assist LLMs in producing more accurate outcomes [23].

Data Preprocessing

After gathering substantial text data to build the pretraining corpus, preprocessing the data is crucial. The process includes eliminating noisy, redundant, unnecessary, and poisonous materials, since these factors might hurt the functionality and performance of LLMs. Data-Juicer [24], a data processing solution with over 50 processing operators and tools for LLMs, helps with data processing.

Quality Filtering

The two commonly used approaches available in the literature to eliminate low-quality data from the obtained corpus are [1] classifier-based and [2] heuristic-based. In the former method, a selection classifier trained on high-quality texts identifies and filters out low-quality material. These techniques usually include training a binary classifier to predict the quality score of each data example using carefully selected data as positive examples and sample candidate data as negative instances. A classifier-based technique, however, may unintentionally exclude high-quality texts in dialectal, colloquial, and sociolect languages, according to multiple studies, leading to bias in the pretraining corpus and reducing the variety of the corpus.

As a second strategy, heuristic-based techniques filter out low-quality texts using a set of carefully crafted principles. Some of the fundamental techniques are as follows:

- **Language-based filtering:** If an LLM is primarily utilized for work involving such languages, filtering text in other languages is possible.

- **Metric-based filtering:** Unnatural sentences, such as perplexity, can be identified and eliminated using evaluation metrics concerning the produced texts.
- **Statistic-based filtering:** To gauge text quality and weed out low-quality data, statistical characteristics of a corpus, such as sentence length, symbol-to-word ratio, and punctuation distribution, can be used.
- **Keyword-based filtering:** A particular set of keywords can be utilized to identify and remove distracting or unnecessary text elements, such as HTML tags, hyperlinks, and boilerplates.

Deduplication

Duplication in à corpus will decrease the variety of LM, leading to an unstable training process and impairing model performance [25]. Therefore, the pretraining corpus has to be deduplicated. In particular, deduplication can occur at various levels of granularity, such as datasets, documents, and sentences. First, as they might promote repeating patterns in language modeling, low-quality sentences with repeated words and phrases should be eliminated [26]. The present methodology commonly uses the overlap ratio of surface characteristics between documents at the document level to identify and eliminate duplicate documents with identical contents. Additionally, eliminating any potential duplicate texts from the training set is essential to eliminate the overlap between the training and assessment sets and avoid dataset contamination.

Privacy

Pretraining text data is mainly sourced from websites, which may contain user-generated content containing private or sensitive information, raising the possibility of privacy violations [27]. As a result, the pretraining corpus must have its Personally Identifiable Information (PII) removed. Using rule-based techniques can be eliminated straightforwardly and efficiently. Moreover, researchers discovered that the pretraining corpus's duplicate PII data is why LLMs are susceptible to privacy attacks. Deduplication can lessen privacy problems.

Tokenization

Another essential phase in the preparation of data is tokenization. Its goal is to divide unprocessed text into sequences of discrete tokens fed into LLMs. Word-based tokenization is the prevalent strategy in classic NLP research [28, 29], as it aligns more with human language comprehension. Word-based tokenization leads to an "out-of-vocabulary" problem, creating an enormous word vocabulary that includes many low-frequency terms and inconsistent segmentation in specific languages. As a result, models are trained using characters as a basic unit necessary to obtain the word representation. Subword tokenizers, such as BytePair Encoding, WordPiece [30], and Unigram tokenization, have recently been extensively employed in Transformer-based language models.

One possible side effect of customized tokenizers is to be mindful while expanding current LLMs. For instance, LLaMA uses a pretraining corpus mainly composed of English texts to train the BPE tokenizer. As a result, the generated vocabulary may need to be more capable of interpreting non-English data, such as Chinese texts, which require a more extended inference latency [31]. Creating appropriate scheduling techniques for multi-source data after data preprocessing is crucial to providing an effective LLM for pretraining. Fig. (**2**) illustrates the data scheduling for pretraining LLMs.

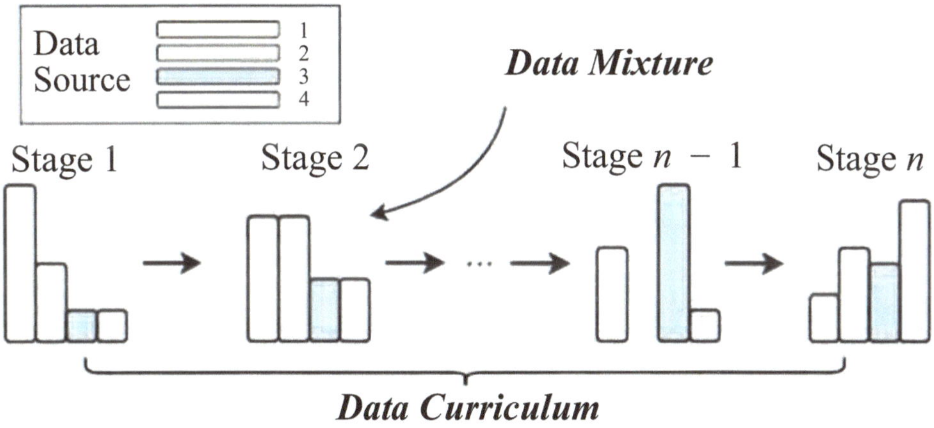

Fig. (2). An example of data scheduling for LLM pretraining [16].

Creating appropriate scheduling techniques for multi-source data after data preprocessing is crucial to providing an effective LLM for pretraining. The two critical factors for data scheduling are the percentage of each data source and the planning of the sequence of data sources.

A. Data Mixture: Since creating specific capacities for LLMs is directly linked to each type of data source, it is crucial to establish an appropriate distribution for combining various data. The data mixture can be locally adjusted to various proportions at different locations. A summary of popular methods for determining an efficient data mixture is as follows:

- **Increasing the diversity of data sources:** Boosting the downstream performance of LLMs requires more significant heterogeneity in data sources. The authors in a study [32] have pre-trained LLMs with carefully selected datasets and carried out ablation experiments by eliminating each data source one at a time to investigate the impact of various data sources. Removing data sources with high heterogeneity, such as websites, has a significant detrimental effect on LLM's performance.

- **Optimizing data mixtures**: Pretraining data that either have a higher closeness in the feature space or have beneficial impacts on the performance of downstream tasks can be chosen based on the desired downstream tasks. Additionally, DoReMi [33] trains a small reference model with initial domain weights provided to lessen the dependence on target tasks. Subsequently, it trains a second small proxy model by weighting the domains where the most significant differences in probability between the two models are detected. Ultimately, a much bigger LLM is trained using the learned domain weights of the proxy model. A more straightforward method is to train many tiny language models with various data combinations and then choose the combination of data that produces the best results. Nonetheless, this method relies on the premise that tiny models will share skills or behaviors with large models when trained similarly, which may not always hold in real-world scenarios.

Data Curriculum: Arranging the sequence for pretraining data sent to LLMs is crucial, even after data mixture preparation. A study [34] indicates that when learning a particular skill, studying in a skillset sequence (basic skills → target skill) is sometimes a better method than learning directly from a corpus that focuses on the target skill. In line with curriculum learning, the data curriculum has been put out and is frequently employed in the pretraining of models. Its goal is to arrange various components of pretraining material for LLMs in a predetermined sequence, such as beginning with simple, broad instances and gradually adding more complex, specialized ones. It may describe the pretraining adaptive adjustment of data proportions for various sources.

For instance, CodeLLaMA was created based on LLaMA 2 to enhance code creation while maintaining natural language comprehension abilities in LLMs. Another offering from CodeLLaMA is a version specifically tailored to a particular programming language, CodeLLaMA-Python [35].

ARCHITECTURE

Fig. (**3**) illustrates three standard architectures used in LLMs. The three primary components of the architecture are the encoder-decoder, the causal decoder, and the prefix decoder.

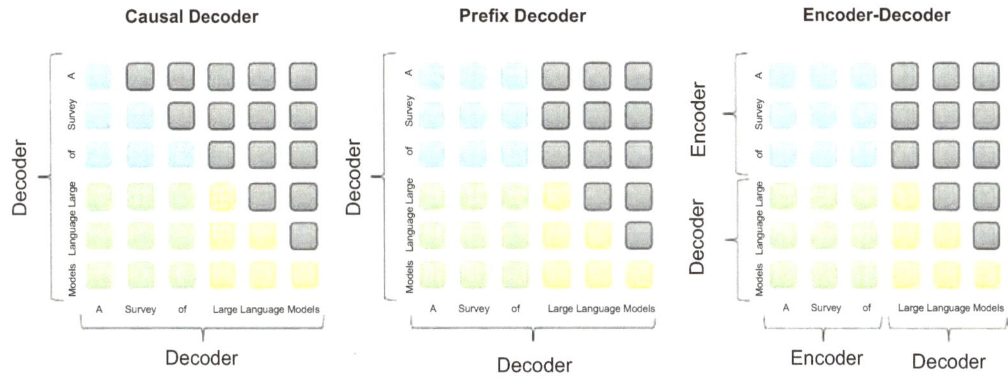

Fig. (3). A comparison of three popular architectures' attention patterns [16].

Encoder-decoder Architecture: The encoder-decoder architecture [36] consists of two stacks of transformer blocks that function as the encoder and decoder, respectively. The encoder uses stacked multi-head self-attention layers to construct its latent representations to encode the input sequence. The decoder then applies cross-attention to these representations and generates the target sequence autoregressively. Encoder-decoder PLMs have demonstrated efficacy on various NLP tasks. Only a few LLMs, such as Flan-T5, have been developed using the encoder-decoder design.

Causal Decoder Architecture: The unidirectional attention mask is incorporated into the causal decoder architecture to ensure that each input token can only focus on itself and the tokens that came before it. The decoder processes the input and output tokens in the same way. The GPT-series models [37] are built on the causal-decoder architecture and serve as representative language models of this architecture.

Prefix Decoder Architecture: The prefix decoder architecture, also known as the non-causal decoder, modifies the causal decoders' masking technique to allow for the performance of unidirectional focus solely on created tokens and bidirectional attention over prefix tokens. The prefix decoders can thus, similarly to the encoder-decoder design, bidirectionally encode the prefix sequence and autoregressively anticipate the output tokens individually while sharing the same parameters. To accelerate convergence, it is practicable to train causal decoders repeatedly and then transform them into prefix decoders, as in the case of U-PaLM, developed from PaLM, rather than starting from scratch with pretraining.

LARGE LANGUAGE MODEL IN HEALTHCARE

While LLMs have demonstrated remarkable performance in various Natural Language Processing tasks, their effectiveness in specialized tasks is restricted [38]. General language maintenance specialists need help understanding technical jargon and providing well-reasoned replies when they need domain-specific expertise. Furthermore, the general and professional corpora differ significantly, which makes it harder for LLMs to perform effectively in biological or clinical activities. Specialized LLMs are being developed to address the above-discussed limitations and improve expertise in specific domains.

Biomedical Text Mining (BioBERT) [39] is the pre-trained model used for biomedical text mining. The model was first trained on English-language and then finetuned on a large biomedical corpus from PubMed. Instead of honing the generic BERT model, SCIBERT was pre-trained using the Semantic Scholar corpora comprising 82% biomedical publications and 18% computer science literature. Using a schema akin to SCIBERT, PubMedBERT was created with just corpora obtained from PubMed. In biomedical NLP tasks, BioBERT outperformed SCIBERT and PubMedBERT compared to BERT. There are a few therapeutic applications for these biological language models.

ClinicalBERT was created using the MIMIC-III data set based on the BERT and BioBERT architectures. A comprehensive collection of domain-specific information of over 40,000 critical care patients is included in MIMIC-III [40]. ClinicalBERT fared better than BERT and BioBERT on various medical NLP tasks, suggesting that LLMs may be optimized for specific domains by utilizing clinical corpora. GatorTron [41], a transformer model, is pre-trained with more than 90 billion words of text from Wikipedia, PubMed articles, and deidentified clinical notes at the University of Florida Health. The model was trained on 8.9 billion clinical parameters, making it one of the largest pre-trained models.

Furthermore, developing LLMs' communication skills has encouraged innovation in the medical field. The PaLM performance was maximized through instruction prompt adjustment to create a chatbot, Med-PaLM [42], for healthcare. The outcome of further research and development at Google is Med-PaLM 2, which is said to outperform ChatGPT and reach state-of-the-art performance on USMLE problems. Based on LLaMA, ChatDoctor is an open-source chatbot designed for the healthcare industry that is finetuned using 100,000 patient-physician talks [43]. This model demonstrated notable gains in comprehending patients' requirements and providing correct advice. Comparably, another open-source chatbot for healthcare, Baize-healthcare, is built on LLaMA and has been optimized with the help of the MedQuAD data set, which contains 46,867 medical dialogues. These models demonstrate the creation of conversation models in healthcare.

While broad LLMs are doing quite well and developing quickly, domain-specific models can still be the best option for some jobs. Future research might focus on prompt-tuning or finetuning these generic LLMs instead of building domain-specific models from the ground up to maximize performance in specific tasks. The skills of decentralized researchers worldwide can be improved by utilizing larger open-source base models and newer technologies. These researchers can then refine LLMs to achieve better performance in clinical work. Tailored LLMs can be developed to perform specific, well-defined tasks, minimizing errors and optimizing therapeutic use through custom adjustments. Whether created from the ground up or refined *via* preexisting models, LLM apps will advance in sophistication and start to influence practitioners and patients significantly.

The excitement surrounding LLMs in the healthcare industry is due to their ability to improve patient care. The healthcare industry expects to see more creative and valuable uses of this technology as LLMs develop. It is important to analyze the hazards and limits associated with using LLMs in the healthcare industry. Examples include vulnerability to security breaches and prejudice. It is imperative to carefully examine LLMs' dangers and limits before applying them in healthcare settings. The popularity of LLMs in healthcare can be attributed to the following factors [44]

1. **The increasing availability of data:** Large datasets of biological and medical literature are readily available to train LLMs. The healthcare sector is producing more data than ever before, which makes it feasible to train LLMs that will enhance patient care.
2. **The decreasing cost of computation:** Processing power prices have gradually declined for many years. As a result, large-scale LLM deployment and training are now feasible.
3. **The increasing demand for personalized healthcare services:** Patients call for more individualized treatment catered to their specific requirements. Personalized treatment regimens and recommendations may be created using LLMs, leading to better patient results.
4. **The potential to improve efficiency and accuracy:** LLMs automate many processes in the healthcare industry, like appointment scheduling and report generation, freeing medical staff members to concentrate on patient care. Additionally, LLMs can increase the precision of diagnosis and therapy.

5. **Personalized Learning Experiences:** Healthcare workers may benefit from customized learning experiences created by LLMs, which help them stay current on the latest medical research and best practices.
6. **Automated Administrative Tasks:** LLMs are skilled at automating report production and appointment scheduling, two administrative duties in the healthcare industry. Thanks to this technology, healthcare workers are free to focus on patient care.

APPLICATION AREAS IN HEALTHCARE

Fig. (**4**) illustrates a typical healthcare patient journey. Pre-consultation is the process by which patients sign up for a consultation or undergo screening. Diagnosis is the process by which patients receive a diagnosis, which includes an examination, a consultation, and any necessary follow-up investigations. Management is the process by which patients receive prescription medications, patient education and counseling, and reimbursement for medical bills. At every one of these patient journey contact points, LLMs have the potential to improve the patient experience.

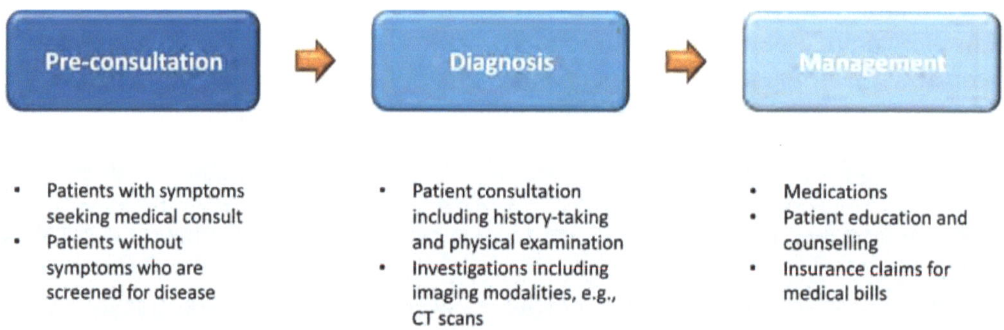

Fig. (4). Implementing big language models within a patient's treatment process [43]

Pre-consultation

By integrating with cloud services, LLMs can help with patient triage and resource allocation. The application over the cloud can suggest that patients with particular medical subspecialties should schedule an appointment [44], reducing medical resource waste by giving patients a framework for recommendations on where to obtain the proper medical review. Additionally, LLMs can be combined with telemedicine services or remote diagnostic systems to improve access to treatment for patients with mobility issues or geographic restrictions. For people in distant areas like sub-Saharan Africa, LLMs can serve as real-time self-assessment tools using mobile platforms such as SMS. This tool facilitated prompt access to healthcare through the evaluation of tropical illness symptoms, the provision of medical advice, and the suggestion of a likely diagnosis. Using extra data such as drug lists, comorbidities, and risk factors, LLMs can enhance predictions about a patient's medical history and evaluate their symptoms.

Diagnosis

In addition to being crucial for diagnosis, patient consultation, particularly the initial visit, is essential for establishing the cornerstone of the patient-physician relationship. Nevertheless, clinical practice is frequently overbooked, resulting in little time for individual patient consultations. Using LLMs, medical practitioners can be provided with a detailed analysis of an electronic health record that might be critical for diagnosing an illness. Additionally, it makes for a more thorough and effective consultation, frees the doctor to spend more time interacting with patients, and improves patient satisfaction.

Adjunctive studies are frequently needed throughout the diagnostic procedure to validate the diagnosis and bolster clinical suspicion. In some clinical settings, LLMs can act as clinical decision-support systems, assisting doctors in choosing the most suitable radiological tests [45] and reducing needless strain on the capacity of currently available resources, particularly in public hospitals or low-resource environments where technical support and imaging modalities are few.

Deep learning models, along with Computer-aided Diagnostic (CAD) systems, can lead to the efficient and highly accurate interpretation of various medical imaging modalities for diagnosing and categorizing diseases. Integrating LLMs into CAD systems may improve the interpretability of the model and promote the adoption of current diagnostic procedures. The physicians can learn new information or find imaging biomarkers of illness throughout the process.

Management

A multidisciplinary approach is necessary for optimal management, with a growing focus on people-centered healthcare, enabling patients to accept responsibility for their well-being and participate in the process [46]. Treatment success depends significantly on medication adherence, often attributed to patient education and support. Including patients in patient education programs may improve adherence and motivate them to take charge of their health. LLMs may make customized patient education possible, increasing comprehension and involvement. Macy, an AI pharmacist with ChatGPT integrated into a photorealistic animated avatar, recently demonstrated the ability to provide a video prescription consultation containing important information, including medicine dose and frequency, safety measures, and warning signs to look out for, all organized in simple language. Even if it is purely experimental, the fact that it was created in less than 30 minutes and for very little money shows how LLMs have the potential to transform patient education and other fields.

Additionally, LLMs can produce instructional materials for patients at the right level, including medication counseling, lifestyle adjustments, and counseling following treatment, making it possible to explain complicated medical jargon to people in a way that is easy to comprehend while still being acceptable and effective. For instance, LLMs may be applied to autocomplete jobs involving text simplification, which suggests the user write basic phrases to follow the physician's written words, simplifying medical reports with a lot of jargon [47]. This allows the doctor to guarantee the information's quality and accuracy while speeding up the text simplification process and maintaining control over the translated content.

Managing individuals with mental health issues requires multimodal and interdisciplinary treatments. In addition to improving patient compliance and fulfilling the clinical requirement for access to mental care services and treatment, LLMs help mitigate the scarcity of medical practitioners. SERMO [48] helps patients with mental health issues better manage negative thoughts. Based on the user's text inputs, it automatically determines the type of emotion and suggests mindfulness exercises or activities appropriate for the particular feeling.

Medical Education

Besides their patient-centered uses, lifelong learning modules have great potential to transform medical research and education. Current LLMs have demonstrated their ability to pass undergraduate and graduate medical exams. Additionally, the reasons for the answers that ChatGPT produced for the USMLE were highly concordant and provided fresh perspectives. Students can easily follow along because of the explanations' logical flow and deductive reasoning supported by further material. Additionally, ChatGPT can offer creative and original mnemonics to help with memorization. LLMs' interactive interfaces can enhance student-directed learning, as students have shown that they favor the Socratic method of instruction over didactic lectures.

LLMs can increase the productivity of research article writing by automating processes, including creating content, conducting a literature review, and providing guidance on formatting and writing style for manuscripts [49]. LLMs can link patients with possible clinical trial opportunities that meet inclusion and exclusion criteria and are pertinent to their problems, making it easier to find study subjects and giving patients access to ground-breaking therapies that they might not otherwise have or cannot afford.

CHALLENGES OF LLMS IN HEALTHCARE

Data Privacy

The possibility of leaking sensitive and private patient data is a challenge in applying and validating LLMs with real-world clinical patient information. Adversarial attacks, for example, efficiently retrieved the training data for an LLM GPT-2. Training data, such as personally identifiable information and Internet Relay Chat logs, was collected verbatim using structured queries by GPT-2. Furthermore, several algorithms showed the potential to re-identify these individuals even after secretly removing critical patient health information [50]. Pseudonymization or filtering patient identification, differential privacy, and data extraction attacks for LLM audits are potential approaches to lessen these difficulties.

Questionable Credibility and Accuracy of Information

The dubious integrity and authenticity of the material produced by LLMs have drawn criticism from several quarters. Open-domain generic LLMs may have inadequate contextual setting generalization or run the danger of propagating false information from open internet sources. Trivial guessing behaviors seen in LLMs have been called the "hallucination effect" [51]. Human monitoring and extra quality controls are crucial in guaranteeing precision and quality assurance of the produced material, even with its ability as a teaching tool and information resource for the medical community, patients, and medical students.

Data Bias

LLMs are trained on large, varied datasets that are commonly skewed. Consequently, bias based on factors like gender, race, and socioeconomic status may be reinforced and amplified in the information produced by LLMs. These biases are particularly harmful in the healthcare industry since unequal treatment can exacerbate existing differences in mortality and morbidity. An LLM that is less skilled in detecting skin cancer in people with darker skin tones, for instance, may be produced by research on skin cancer that mainly includes participants with light complexion, resulting in incorrect diagnoses, postponed or ineffective treatments, and increased health inequities. When minority groups are absent from training data, LLMs may amplify preexisting biases and produce unreliable outcomes. For LLMs, transitioning to equitable artificial intelligence and fighting against prejudice will be formidable challenges [52].

Interpretability of LLMs

Adoption into clinical practice is hampered by the decision-making process of the interpretability issue with LLMs [53]. The majority of LLM-generated replies need explanations or citations for supporting data. Creswell et al. [54] proposed a multi-step reasoning framework for selection inference to increase interpretability. It generates several haphazard reasoning stages leading to the final generated response. A comprehensible linear framework for text categorization was trained using an additional approach that leverages step-by-step instructions, or chain-o--thought prompting, for knowledge graph extraction, involving presenting the entities and relationships extracted from the unprocessed source text in an organized manner. Another helpful feature may be uncertainty-aware LLM applications, which increase user confidence in suggested LLM applications by reporting confidence scores of produced replies or using various weights for input data.

Roles of LLMs

Another potential difficulty is determining the role and identification of LLMs in clinical practice and scientific research. Among the queries that might arise are: Is AI capable of being a doctor or a researcher? Is the material produced by the AI its fault? How can I tell the difference between writing produced by AI and human writers? What should be done when doctors hold opinions that differ from AI's? LLMs can create fake material. Hence, excessive use must be avoided [55]. Physician monitoring is still necessary to guarantee that the generated information is correct and therapeutically relevant, even if LLMs are capable of self-improvement.

Deployment of LLMs

The open-source nature of LLaMA makes it easier to install LLMs on devices with limited resources, such as Raspberry Pi systems, laptops, and phones. Alpaca's LLaMA-based finetuning makes it possible to create models with performance that is on par with GPT-3.5 in a matter of hours and at a price of less than US$600 [56], reducing the cost of training high-performing customized language models. Creating and implementing several safeguards to utilize LLMs for the intended goals and to lower the hazards connected with their abuse is imperative. These involve the development of strict terms of use and deployment guidelines, as well as technological methods for removing offensive and sensitive information. Using such procedures makes it possible to properly manage the potential risks of LLM deployment on tiny personal devices.

Clinical Domain-specific LLMs

Without question, LLMs are making a big difference in the healthcare industry. Pre-consultation, diagnosis, Management, medical education, and medical writing are the only fields that will encounter revolutionary shifts due to LLM growth. In this context, it is crucial to understand that various medical professions will face multiple obstacles when implementing LLMs in actual clinical settings [57]. For instance, significant differences in the kind and caliber of data between domains may exist. Furthermore, the many activities and application scenarios that LLMs might use will result in disparities in the criteria that clinical practitioners require. Because of this, we should be aware of the differences across clinical specializations while implementing LLMs in clinical settings and adapt as necessary to the particular application scenarios.

CONCLUSION

Healthcare will significantly shift, and LLMs will play a significant role in this industry. Retraining the use of medical databases or generic LLMs to finetune might help develop strategies to improve the usability of LLMs for healthcare. Additionally, multimodal LLMs can feature fusion using various data sources, including tabular and visual data, which leads to even greater performance than humans. Even though there are many advantages to using LLMs, it is essential to acknowledge that the content created cannot be solely the responsibility of LLMs. To prevent any potential harm, it is crucial to thoroughly evaluate anything AI generates. Reducing the bar for LLM deployments means that there is more time to focus on improving deployment requirements. To better assist clinical decision-making, efforts should be made to encourage the incorporation of LLMs in medicine, strengthen human-machine collaboration, and enhance LLM interpretability in clinical contexts. Physicians may optimize the advantages of AI while minimizing possible hazards and improving patient outcomes by utilizing LLMs as an auxiliary tool. Ultimately, the cooperation of administrators, patients, data scientists, doctors, and regulatory agencies will be necessary to integrate LLMs into healthcare effectively.

REFERENCES

[1] Miller N, Oldham G, Pinker S. The language instinct: How the mind creates language. Antioch Rev 1994; 52(3): 534.
[http://dx.doi.org/10.2307/4613021]

[2] Turing AM. Computing machinery and intelligence. In: Epstein Robert and Roberts G and BG, editor. Parsing the Turing Test: Philosophical and Methodological Issues in the Quest for the Thinking Computer [Internet]. Dordrecht: Springer Netherlands; 2009. p. 23–65.
[http://dx.doi.org/10.1007/978-1-4020-6710-5_3]

[3] Gao J, Lin C-Y. Introduction to the special issue on statistical language modeling. ACM Trans Asian Lang Inf Process 2004; 3(2): 87-93.

[http://dx.doi.org/10.1145/1034780.1034781]

[4] Zhai CX. Statistical Language Models for Information Retrieval. Springer Cham 2009. [http://dx.doi.org/10.1007/978-3-031-02130-5]

[5] Brants T, Popat AC, Xu P, Och FJ, Dean J. Large language models in machine translation. In: Eisner J, editor. Proceedings of the 2007 Joint Conference on Empirical Methods in Natural Language Processing and Computational Natural Language Learning (EMNLP-CoNLL). Prague, Czech Republic: Association for Computational Linguistics; 2007. p. 858–67. Available from: https://aclanthology.org/D07-1090/

[6] Mikolov T, Karafiát M, Burget L, Cernocký J, Khudanpur S. Recurrent neural network based language model. 2010.

[7] Bengio Y, Ducharme R, Vincent P, *et al.* A Neural Probabilistic Language Model. Vol. 3. J Mach Learn Res 2003.

[8] Peters ME, Neumann M, Gardner M, Clark C, Lee K, Zettlemoyer L. Deep contextualized word representations. In: Proceedings of NAACL-HLT 2018 [Internet]. 2018. p. 2227–37. Available from: http://allennlp.org/elmo10.18653/v1/N18-1202

[9] Radford A, Wu J, Child R, Luan D, Amodei D, Sutskever I. Language Models are Unsupervised Multitask Learners [Internet]. Available from: https://github.com/codelucas/newspaper

[10] Kaplan J, McCandlish S, Henighan T, *et al.* Scaling laws for neural language models. arXiv [cs.LG]. 2020; arXiv:2001.08361. [http://dx.doi.org/10.48550/arXiv.2001.08361]

[11] Hoffmann J, Borgeaud S, Mensch A, *et al.* Training compute-optimal large language models. Proceedings of the 36th International Conference on Neural Information Processing Systems 2024.

[12] Taylor R, Kardas M, Cucurull G, *et al.* Galactica: A large language model for science. arXiv [cs.CL]. 2022; arXiv:2211.09085. [http://dx.doi.org/10.48550/arXiv.2211.09085]

[13] Wei J, Bosma M, Zhao VY, Guu K, Yu AW, Lester B, et al. FINETUNED LANGUAGE MODELS ARE ZERO-SHOT LEARNERS Closed-Book QA [Internet]. 2022. Available from: https://github.com/google-research/flan

[14] Schick T, Dwivedi-Yu J, Dessì R, *et al.* Toolformer: Language models can teach themselves to use tools. arXiv [cs.CL]. 2023; arXiv:2302.04761. [http://dx.doi.org/10.48550/arXiv.2302.04761]

[15] Brown T, Mann B, Ryder N, *et al.* Language models are few-shot learners. arXiv [cs.LG]. 2020; arXiv:2005.14165. [http://dx.doi.org/10.48550/arXiv.2005.14165]

[16] Zhao WX, Zhou K, Li J, Tang T, Wang X, Hou Y, et al. A Survey of Large Language Models. ArXiv [Internet]. 2023;1–124. Available from: http://arxiv.org/abs/2303.18223

[17] Chowdhery A, Narang S, Devlin J, *et al.* PaLM: Scaling language modeling with Pathways. arXiv [cs.CL]. 2022; arXiv:2204.02311. [http://dx.doi.org/10.48550/arXiv.2204.02311]

[18] Zhang S, Roller S, Goyal N, *et al.* OPT: Open Pre-trained Transformer Language Models. arXiv [cs.CL]. 2022; arXiv:2205.01068. [http://dx.doi.org/10.48550/arXiv.2205.01068]

[19] Zhu Y, Kiros R, Zemel R, *et al.* Aligning Books and Movies: Towards Story-Like Visual Explanations by Watching Movies and Reading Books In: 2015 IEEE International Conference on Computer Vision (ICCV). Los Alamitos, CA, USA: IEEE Computer Society 2015; pp. 19-27. Internet Available from: https://doi.ieeecomputersociety.org/ [http://dx.doi.org/10.1109/ICCV.2015.11]

[20] Gao L, Biderman S, Black S, *et al.* The Pile: An 800GB Dataset of Diverse Text for Language Modeling. 2020 Dec 31 Available from: http://arxiv.org/abs/2101.00027

[21] Li X, Yao Y, Jiang X, *et al.* FLM-101B: An Open LLM and How to Train It with $100K Budget. 2023 Sep 7. Available from: http://arxiv.org/abs/2309.03852

[22] Saier T, Krause J, Färber M. unarXive 2022: All arXiv Publications Pre-Processed for NLP, Including Structured Full-Text and Citation Network. 2023 Mar 27 Available from: http://arxiv.org/abs/2303.14957

[23] Madaan A, Zhou S, Alon U, Yang Y, Neubig G. Language Models of Code are Few-Shot Commonsense Learners. 2022 Oct 13; Available from: http://arxiv.org/abs/2210.07128 [http://dx.doi.org/10.18653/v1/2022.emnlp-main.90]

[24] Chen D, Huang Y, Ma Z, *et al.* Data-Juicer: A One-Stop Data Processing System for Large Language Models. Proc ACM SIGMOD Int Conf Manag Data 2024; 120-34. [http://dx.doi.org/10.1145/3626246.3653385]

[25] Hernandez D, Brown T, Conerly T, *et al.* Scaling Laws and Interpretability of Learning from Repeated Data. 2022 May 20; Available from: http://arxiv.org/abs/2205.10487

[26] Holtzman A, Buys J, Du L, Forbes M, Choi Y. The Curious Case of Neural Text Degeneration. In: 8th International Conference on Learning Representations, ICLR 2020,Addis Ababa, Ethiopia, April 26-30, 2020 [Internet]. OpenReview.net; 2020 Available from: https://openreview.net/forum?id=rygGQyrFvH

[27] Carlini N, Tramèr F, Lee K, *et al.* Extracting Training Data from Large Language Models [Internet]. Available from: https://www.usenix.org/conference/usenixsecurity21/presentation/carlini-extracting

[28] Laurençon H, Saulnier L, Wang T, *et al.* The BigScience ROOTS Corpus: A 1.6TB Composite Multilingual Dataset. In: 36th Conference on Neural Information Processing Systems (NeurIPS 2022) Track on Datasets and Benchmarks [Internet]. 2022. p. 2–18. Available from: https://bigscience.huggingface.co/

[29] Lafferty JD, McCallum A, Pereira FCN. Conditional Random Fields: Probabilistic Models for Segmenting and Labeling Sequence Data. Proceedings of the Eighteenth International Conference on Machine Learning 2001; 282-9.

[30] Schuster M, Nakajima K. Japanese and Korean voice search. 2012 IEEE International Conference on Acoustics, Speech and Signal Processing (ICASSP) 2012; 5149-2. [http://dx.doi.org/10.1109/ICASSP.2012.6289079]

[31] Wu Y, Schuster M, Chen Z, *et al.* Google's Neural Machine Translation System: Bridging the Gap between Human and Machine Translation. 2016 Sep 26;. Available from: http://arxiv.org/abs/1609.08144

[32] Longpre S, Yauney G, Reif E, *et al.* A Pretrainer's Guide to Training Data: Measuring the Effects of Data Age, Domain Coverage, Quality, & Toxicity. 2023 May 22; Available from: http://arxiv.org/abs/2305.13169

[33] Xie SM, Pham H, Dong X, *et al.* DoReMi: Optimizing Data Mixtures Speeds Up Language Model Pretraining. 2023 May 17; Available from: http://arxiv.org/abs/2305.10429

[34] Chen MF, Roberts N, Bhatia K, *et al.* Skill-it! A Data-Driven Skills Framework for Understanding and Training Language Models. 2023 Jul 26; Available from: http://arxiv.org/abs/2307.14430

[35] Rozière B, Gehring J, Gloeckle F, *et al.* Code Llama: Open Foundation Models for Code. 2023 Aug 24. Available from: http://arxiv.org/abs/2308.12950

[36] Vaswani A, Brain G, Shazeer N, *et al.* Attention Is All You Need. 31st Conference on Neural Information Processing Systems (NIPS 2017) 2017; 1-17.

[37] Openai AR, Openai KN, Openai TS, Openai IS. Improving Language Understanding by Generative

Pretraining [Internet]. Available from: https://gluebenchmark.com/leaderboard

[38] Thirunavukarasu AJ, Hassan R, Mahmood S, *et al.* Trialling a Large Language Model (ChatGPT) in General Practice With the Applied Knowledge Test: Observational Study Demonstrating Opportunities and Limitations in Primary Care. JMIR Med Educ 2023; 9: e46599. [http://dx.doi.org/10.2196/46599] [PMID: 37083633]

[39] Lee J, Yoon W, Kim S, *et al.* BioBERT: a pre-trained biomedical language representation model for biomedical text mining. Bioinformatics 2020; 36(4): 1234-40. [http://dx.doi.org/10.1093/bioinformatics/btz682] [PMID: 31501885]

[40] Johnson AEW, Pollard TJ, Shen L, *et al.* MIMIC-III, a freely accessible critical care database. Sci Data 2016; 3(1): 160035. [http://dx.doi.org/10.1038/sdata.2016.35] [PMID: 27219127]

[41] Yang X, Chen A, PourNejatian N, *et al.* A large language model for electronic health records. npj. Digit Med 2022; 5(1): 1-9. [PMID: 35663827]

[42] Chen S. Potential Applications and Safety of Large Language Models in Healthcare. Interdiscip Humanit Commun Stud [Internet]. 2024; Available from: https://api.semanticscholar.org/CorpusID:269204770 [http://dx.doi.org/10.61173/f578jp05]

[43] Yang R, Tan TF, Lu W, Thirunavukarasu AJ, Ting DSW, Liu N. Large language models in health care: Development, applications, and challenges. Vol. 2, Health Care Science. John Wiley and Sons Inc; 2023. p. 255–63.

[44] Wang J, Zhang G, Wang W, Zhang K, Sheng Y. Cloud-based intelligent self-diagnosis and department recommendation service using Chinese medical BERT. J Cloud Comput (Heidelb) 2021; 10(1): 4. [http://dx.doi.org/10.1186/s13677-020-00218-2]

[45] Shen Y, Heacock L, Elias J, *et al.* ChatGPT and Other Large Language Models Are Double-edged Swords. Vol. 307, Radiology. Radiological Society of North America Inc.; 2023. [http://dx.doi.org/10.1148/radiol.230163]

[46] Organization WH. WHO global strategy on people-centred and integrated health services: interim report. World Health Organization 2015.

[47] Van H, Kauchak D, Leroy G. AutoMeTS: The Autocomplete for Medical Text Simplification. In: Scott D, Bel N, Zong C, editors. Proceedings of the 28th International Conference on Computational Linguistics [Internet]. Barcelona, Spain (Online): International Committee on Computational Linguistics; 2020. p. 1424–34. Available from: https://aclanthology.org/2020.coling-main.122

[48] Denecke K, Vaaheesan S, Arulnathan A. A Mental Health Chatbot for Regulating Emotions (SERMO) - Concept and Usability Test. IEEE Trans Emerg Top Comput 2021; 9(3): 1170-82. [http://dx.doi.org/10.1109/TETC.2020.2974478]

[49] Abou-Hanna JJ, Owens ST, Kinnucan JA, Mian SI, Kolars JC. Resuscitating the Socratic Method: Student and Faculty Perspectives on Posing Probing Questions During Clinical Teaching. Acad Med 2021; 96(1): 113-7. [http://dx.doi.org/10.1097/ACM.0000000000003580] [PMID: 33394663]

[50] Gymrek M, McGuire AL, Golan D, Halperin E, Erlich Y. Identifying Personal Genomes by Surname Inference. Science (80-) [Internet]. 2013;339(6117):321–4. Available from: https://www.science.org/ [http://dx.doi.org/10.1126/science.1229566]

[51] Volovici V, Syn NL, Ercole A, Zhao JJ, Liu N. Steps to avoid overuse and misuse of machine learning in clinical research. Nat Med 2022; 28(10): 1996-9. [http://dx.doi.org/10.1038/s41591-022-01961-6] [PMID: 36097217]

[52] Norori N, Hu Q, Aellen FM, Faraci FD, Tzovara A. Addressing bias in big data and AI for health care: A call for open science. Patterns (N Y) 2021; 2(10): 100347. Available from:

https://www.sciencedirect.com/science/article/pii/S2666389921002026
[http://dx.doi.org/10.1016/j.patter.2021.100347] [PMID: 34693373]

[53] Tjoa E, Guan C. A Survey on Explainable Artificial Intelligence (XAI): Toward Medical XAI. IEEE Trans Neural Netw Learn Syst 2021; 32(11): 4793-813.
[http://dx.doi.org/10.1109/TNNLS.2020.3027314] [PMID: 33079674]

[54] Creswell A, Shanahan M, Higgins I. Selection-Inference: Exploiting Large Language Models for Interpretable Logical Reasoning. 2022;1–33. Available from: http://arxiv.org/abs/2205.09712

[55] Wei J, Wang X, Schuurmans D, *et al.* Chain-of-thought prompting elicits reasoning in large language models. Proceedings of the 36th International Conference on Neural Information Processing Systems 2024.

[56] B. RT and IG and TZ and YD and XL and CG and PL and T. Alpaca: A Strong, Replicable Instruction-Following Model [Internet]. 2024. Available from: https://crfm.stanford.edu/2023/03/13/alpaca.html

[57] Cascella M, Montomoli J, Bellini V, Bignami E. Evaluating the Feasibility of ChatGPT in Healthcare: An Analysis of Multiple Clinical and Research Scenarios. J Med Syst 2023; 47(1): 33.
[http://dx.doi.org/10.1007/s10916-023-01925-4] [PMID: 36869927]

CHAPTER 10

Ethical and Legal Framework for AI in Healthcare

Misha Bahmani[1,*] and **Shobhna Jeet**[2]

[1] *IILM Law School, IILM University, Gurugram, India*

[2] *School of Legal Studies, K. R. Mangalam University, Gurugram, India*

Abstract: The adoption of new technology by a nation plays a vital role in its growth. The use of AI systems in the healthcare sector holds a stronger position with the increasing presence of advanced technology. These systems provide recognition to the processing and analysis stage, where medical data is considered, its pattern is located, and information is gathered. However, there is a high risk involved when any new form of technology is utilized in reality. In society, there is a need to understand the significance of maintaining both ethical and legal aspects when using AI systems. With transformative technology, the livelihood of an individual is impacted. In healthcare, any error in procedures and protocols can lead to disaster. The integration of these systems in medical practice requires an effective legal framework that can safeguard human health. There is a need for training and education sessions for the stakeholders to have awareness of the new technologies' complexities. This chapter will highlight the critical concerns that are required to be taken into focus to maintain privacy and algorithmic transparency. It guides the policy draft makers to consider the moral grounds to ensure accessibility. Since the level of danger is unpredictable, the AI utilization needs to have its limitations. With effective harmonized governance, the adoption of AI will navigate more opportunities and build a landscape that will be beneficial for mankind.

Keywords: AI system, Algorithm, Ethical, Healthcare, Legal framework, Privacy, Technology.

INTRODUCTION

In the field of healthcare, the utilization of AI has been the most recent change that has been introduced. Being under the domain of computer science, AI is expected to make the system more efficient and quicker. With the presence of dedicated algorithms, the aspect of problem-solving and learning has become more approachable. By recognizing the repetitive patterns, the technology is based on drawing conclusions.

* **Corresponding author Misha Bahmani:** IILM Law School, IILM University, Gurugram, India; E-mail: papermisha@gmail.com

Neeraj Gupta, Abdelhameed Ibrahim, Bhavesh Vyas & Shobhna Jeet (Eds.)

With the development in this sector, several applications have been strengthening its performance. For instance, machine learning has been used to perform various roles in this sector. Providing information about the patients from multiple platforms has resulted in the formation of structured data. This has opened the pathway for innovative ideas and the delivery of accurate information. This technology has guided doctors by providing diagnoses and treatment plans, along with estimated predictions. It is beneficial in monitoring and developing medicines. To promote preventive measures, the healthcare sector is focused on updating itself with new innovative AI applications nowadays [1].

To maintain the smooth functioning and effective monitoring of this technology, there is a requirement for an ethical and legal regulatory framework to ensure adequate involvement of AI in healthcare activities [1]. To support the efficiency and accuracy of diagnosis and treatment systems, AI has been a great guide during the COVID-19 pandemic. Post this pandemic, AI has been introduced in the service facility. Unfortunately, the concern arises about patient information confidentiality. There is a requirement to train the employees before taking assistance from any AI system. There is a need to maintain human equity and focus on preventive measures, as there might be errors while operating this system. There is a requirement of liability and responsibility when considering such situations. There is an urgency to have governance for maintaining collaborative steps that address ethical and legal considerations while using these technologies. Data security, appropriate consent, and privacy are essential elements to prevail in ethical AI. These technologies are required to be free from bias, and governance for software and algorithms should be uniformly applied. Also, they need to maintain transparency while addressing social and ethical concerns, which require a protective regulatory framework [2]. To have improved outcomes, research skills, and clinical trial results, AI must be monitored to attain a healthy impact on the environment [3].

The WHO's report has highlighted the principles and considerations that must be followed for ethical reasons. By reflecting on the challenges, this report has determined the gaps that must be addressed to maintain AI standards in the future [4]. It can be a great contributor to achieving sustainability to attain universal health coverage. Despite this, it has been a matter of concern regarding how transnational issues can be taken into consideration. Software utilization and its computing have resulted in various challenges in addressing human health support. To promote the practice of human autonomy and technology accessibility, AI needs to be regulated and monitored adequately. There is a need to invest in healthcare technology to strengthen AI usage in emerging and developed nations. To fight against misleading data, illegal usage of applications, and ineffective health applications, there is a necessity to have ethical and legal parameters to safeguard the dignity, confidentiality, and privacy of an individual as a patient [5]. There is a need to engage in adaptability and interaction with the data while providing this service. Victims of data breaches are required to have preventive mechanisms in place. Effective governance leads to ethical behavior, which results in the development of algorithms that predict and offer help in drug discovery, diagnosis, and operational efficiency. Medical decisions should be human-protective, based on the possibility of providing remedies for healthcare facilities [6]. Human intelligence combined with AI requires the effective development of algorithms and computational methods through which machines can predict accurate data, and this information can be used for achieving determined goals. Healthcare facilities can only be improved when appropriate guidelines are provided by the authorities. To support clinical performance, there is a need to reduce human errors, which requires technology that prevents unforeseeable circumstances. Ethically, there is a necessity to have qualified and trained medical manpower. The liability of prescriptions generated by AI is unclear, which requires stakeholders in this field to be obedient followers of the legislative system in the near future. AI integration in this would require stronger and narrower tasks to be fulfilled properly with effective moral standards and a legitimate approach [7].

Ethical Standards: AI Use in Healthcare

There is a need to understand that sensitivity should be among the primary goals of maintaining AI as a safety tool. Being accessible, it must be ensured that there is no invasion of privacy. Due to its inclusivity, AI is required to be examined. Being non-discriminatory would lower the risk involved. Despite contextual and emotional intelligence, it is required to be user-centric, which will lead to safer AI. AI being responsible could result in attaining sustainability. It is essential that AI ethics be based on these aspects, which would enhance user participation. By maintaining fairness in AI systems, the outcomes will be beneficial in considering societal requirements. The technology can be utilized for users' comfort by understanding their needs. By reflecting on their emotions and needs, one can understand the user's objective in preferring AI systems. Such practices enhance the vital role of prevailing ethical standards when using these systems. With responsible AI developers, the security and integrity of healthcare prevail. The AI models should only be used for authorized purposes and should prevent manipulation. With social values, the AI ecosystem would fulfill societal requirements. With technical support, its performance can be improved and result in the fulfillment of long-term goals. By incorporating ethics into technology implementation, its ecosystem would become equitable and reliable. With an awareness program, AI governance can be ethically formulated. Monitoring will guide AI in its functioning and will fulfill the user's needs. Transparency in this system will safeguard the stakeholders' interest and their users. Personal and sensitive data requires guiding principles that will strengthen security measures and collaborative relations [8].

Human autonomy and well-being promote these systems to be accountable and responsible for organized planning and development. Being user-centric, there is a need to ensure patient privacy and the utilization of technology for welfare purposes only. NATO has emphasized the significance of building a society that is responsible and upgrades itself to fulfill its requirements. These technologies require governance, which can resolve the difficulties. The WHO has initiated an understanding of the significance of equity and protecting human autonomy to prevent and resolve errors in healthcare. The care disparities should be handled with reasonable care and caution. Sensitive data requires security, as patient safety is the foremost concern. There is a need to have a competent algorithm that does not make errors and facilitates better services in clinics and hospitals. The same errors in an algorithm can have a disastrous impact on healthcare. There is a need to develop an optimal trust level to engage the AI system in healthcare. With transparency, healthcare uses algorithms to fulfill the requirements of this sector. Proper data collection, unbiased algorithms, diversity through ethical standards, and training AI systems are beneficial in achieving remote future goals. The risks can be lowered when ethical principles are established and regulations are made for developing these systems in healthcare [9]. By engaging in ethical considerations, AI applications can be effectively utilized in care management, health monitoring, research purposes, diagnostics, and drug discovery [3].

Ethical Challenges

In this busy lifestyle, reliability is among the primary concerns. There is a need to have an environment where controlled equipment is used and treatment is delivered effectively. When making decisions in healthcare, there is no room to commit errors. With the use of new AI, the concern arises when a nondetectable error occurs, and it is unclear who will be considered liable for it. Safety measures must be taken seriously, as any error can lead to unfavorable implications. Concerns arise when there is difficulty in determining the logic set behind an output generated. There are a few AIs that are proprietary and have maintained secrecy in their functioning [10]. However, there are some that have high complexity levels, which are difficult for humans to determine. There is a necessity to maintain validity as these indefinite outcomes would lead to bias and instability [11].

Unfortunately, there have been incidents where the AI that has been used to train the AI systems has been unsatisfactory and deficient in its functioning, resulting in inadequate mapping that leads to unfair and biased effects and a contradictory impact on societal interests. It should be the responsibility of AI developers to provide algorithms that are unbiased and maintain behavioral standards. It must be a collective initiative to maintain focus on safeguarding and protecting individuals with rare diseases and medical conditions. The issues of this population should be addressed properly, and adequate research data is required to be maintained for effective clinical trials. The United Kingdom's parliament notified that this has been one of their major concerns [12]. There is a need to have clarity in maintaining trust in the information provided by AI systems. For instance, while supporting people with chronic illnesses, the AI system is not able to develop a good bond with humans. This may lead to a negative impact affecting their health. Any unmonitored formation of AI can result in flawed consequences [13]. Unfortunately, social isolation may lead to a rise in more worries when human interaction ends. Replacing humans' participation as staff or family visits might have a grievous impact on their physical and mental well-being. As a precautionary measure, there should be limitations imposed by governmental authorities to keep the system updated, keeping in mind the overall growth of society [14]. The patients should not experience unnecessary restrictions that can have a dreadful impact on their decisions. Importantly, professionals belonging to this sector can utilize this system to seek guidance rather than totally depending on it. By performing automatic tasks, there can be a reduction of staff, which will result in a struggle when these systems decline to consider individual requests.

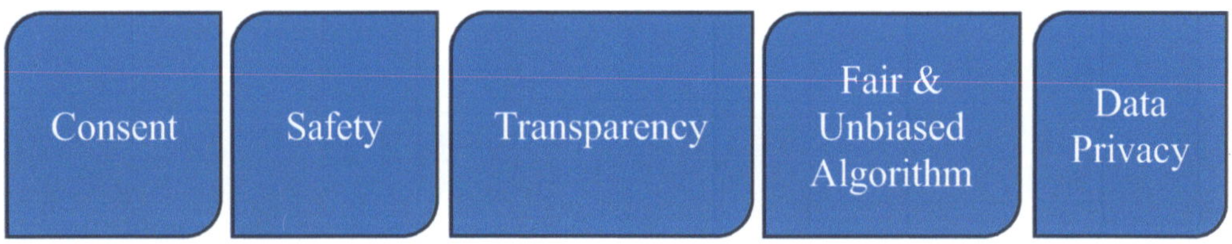

Fig. (1). Ethical standards required.

The figure above, reproduced from Medium, shows the essential requirements for maintaining ethical standards [15]. This shows that despite a technical error and fewer staff being involved in this scenario, the limited number and absence of skilled training will lead to various difficulties. Under a threatening atmosphere, there has been a surge in cybercrimes globally. AI systems are huge targets for getting hacked and spammed [16]. The government should emphasize preparing AI to fight against unethical activities on these platforms. There is a need to have global governance of transformative technologies. National security is the highest priority for maintaining peacekeeping relations. There will be irreparable damage when morals are not maintained when using AI in healthcare [17].

Legal Framework: AI Use in Healthcare

In society, there is a requirement to have legal implications for applying new transformative technologies. Developing AI would make the healthcare system more user-friendly. This will promote preventive and protective measures in the AI ecosystem. Minimizing risks and conducting continuous assessments will make the system reliable for healthcare [8]. Through legal awareness and training efforts, the healthcare sector will be familiarized with the advantages of AI systems. For instance, the FDA has recently expressed its concern about having collaborative initiatives towards promoting innovation and maintaining quality and safety while AI is used for the creation of medical products. It has highlighted the need to consider critical areas to prevail in cybersecurity. Best practices and guidelines need to be uniformly applied for public safety. Through their centers, it emphasizes developing policies for using AI. With effective monitoring and detection of the gaps, there is a necessity to have clarity on where AI is permissible. Developing a methodology to evaluate AI algorithms fairly is a crucial requirement [18]. With the surge in technology, AI tends to grow, which requires proper mapping to preserve humanity. The framework should emphasize on legal use of data, which is built on diversity and equality. AI assists in performing various tasks and provides a neutral outcome without any bias. With harmonized standards in ethical and lawful indications, its ecosystem in healthcare would lead to technological and societal progress for the well-being of humanity [8]. The WHO has stated that AI should be sustainable and respond to user requirements. The laws should be confined to healthcare for establishing AI systems, as their lawful nature allows them to deal with data preservation and cybersecurity. The purpose of these systems is to safeguard AI developers, clinicians, and patients [19].

Legal Challenges

There is a need to focus on the legal responsibility when AI systems are introduced in a nation through its legal system. To regulate AI, global laws should reflect on the security and concealment of personal data. There is a necessity to impose stricter laws that will restrict the transfer of information. There is a requirement to have comprehensive laws to regulate AI systems worldwide. Errors and losses occur when AI systems are used without human participation. Issues of infringement and ownership highlight the need for laws that monitor intellectual property [20]. There is a need to maintain commercial protection of these systems and data-based healthcare facilities. The user needs to be dependent on exemption grounds for IPR infringement when the data is non-licensed or non-owned [21]. To achieve improved health outcomes, there must be a need to have clarity about their governance. The rules should be clearly stated to impose liability when AI systems make errors. AI usage must gain legal acceptance to promote digital health. In emerging nations, there is a need for larger clinical quality datasets, which would be beneficial in providing training and validation for AI [22]. The legislative concern should propose stricter legal policies for AI connections to sustain privacy, data preservation, and an active governing framework. This can be clearly seen from the figure below that, in the legal framework suggested by Amini *et al.*, there is a necessity to have a better implication of policy in the AI domain [23].

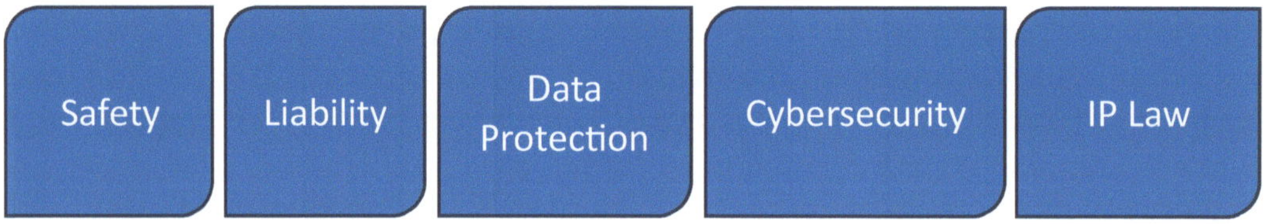

Fig. (2). Legal framework required.

This suggests that there is a need to focus on the human rights aspect when implementing an AI system. Unfortunately, there is a huge risk of misuse of health data, as nowadays, there is insufficient data that is not beneficial in the formation of the algorithm, and due to this, the absence of a regulatory framework for maintaining uniform records can have a rigorous impact on developing nations [24].

Requirements in AI

There is a need to have an ethical standard based on genuine concern, which provides substantive guidance to execute AI [25]. A proper framework is required for monitoring and regulating researchers who are formulating AI systems in healthcare. Globally, there is a need for uniform and standardized principles in relation to AI. The medical data is maintained using AI systems, although it has its limitations, particularly in the involvement of these technologies in clinical practice in some nations. The reasons for implementing this limitation require proper explanation [26].

There is a need to maintain transparency and a human-centric approach when using AI systems in healthcare. The focus must be on the interpretation of various AI systems to develop faith and trust in this practice. It is significant to understand the reasoning behind the decisions made by healthcare professionals. Responsible actions are required to be taken to overcome unwanted challenges in the future. For efficient healthcare delivery and treatment, it is vital that there be fair and unbiased AI involvement in healthcare. In order to have an outcome, the AI systems must be nondiscriminatory. Every characteristic in a group or individual has its significance, which requires adequate assistance to attain equitable results. The dependency on limited generalization can lead to bias, which can have an adverse impact on healthcare [8]. Some AI systems have been created from datasets that are specific in nature, and due to this, the data falls under the category of nonexistence [27]. To understand the human perspective, AI systems must be based on all the parameters to understand the pattern. Unfortunately, AI systems do not understand human common sense and solely rely on their models to cover up the gaps. It struggles to adjust to real-life circumstances and can lead to errors. The focus needs to be on cost and breaking language barriers to implement effective AI systems [8].

Every stage is required to be based on lawful and ethical guidelines to uphold justice. These guidelines require formalization, which can guide the AI developers. There is a need to have proper monitoring of these guidelines to safeguard the interests of both individuals and groups. This will result in effective governance of these systems. With detailed structure and technical assistance, AI systems can maintain their ethnicity in healthcare [28]. There must be responsible usage of these technologies to maintain the quality and safety measures in the creation of medical products.

CONCLUDING REMARKS

With regard to ethical implications, the data can be secure and utilized adequately by maintaining diversity. To fulfill individual interests, these dimensions would encourage transparency by safeguarding their privacy. To avoid risks, its usage should be based on societal welfare and development. The AI support should be based on human interest while using applications. A harmonized legal and ethical framework would encourage the creation of new technologies to be based on the grounds of accountability and standardization [8]. AI developers should focus on fairness and a solution-based approach. Human values are required to be intact in order to achieve social and individual good. Safety and choice should be considered seriously as ethical principles in AI systems [28]. With uniform AI governance guidelines, the developers should highlight fulfilling futuristic societal requirements [8]. There is a need to have a regulatory framework to ensure appropriate data accessibility and distribution. Currently, AI health applications are an understudied area, which reflects the necessity to understand data owner rights. By maintaining an equitable approach while using AI in healthcare, sustainability and determined goals can be achieved [23, 3].

REFERENCES

[1] Anishchenko MA, Gidenko I, Kaliman M, Polyvaniuk V, Demianchuk YV. Artificial intelligence in medicine: Legal, ethical and social aspects. Acta Bioeth 2023; 29(1): 63-72. Available from: https://actabioethica.uchile.cl/index.php/AB/article/view/70910

[http://dx.doi.org/10.4067/S1726-569X2023000100063]

[2] Obasa AE, Palk AC. Responsible application of artificial intelligence in health care. S Afr J Sci 2023; 119(5/6): 14889.
[http://dx.doi.org/10.17159/sajs.2023/14889] [PMID: 39328370]

[3] Bouderhem R. Shaping the future of AI in healthcare through ethics and governance. Humanit Soc Sci Commun 2024; 11(1): 416.
[http://dx.doi.org/10.1057/s41599-024-02894-w]

[4] World Health Organization. Ethics and governance of artificial intelligence for health: WHO guidance [Online]. 2021 [cited 2025 Jan 22]. Available from: https://iris.who.int/bitstream/handle/10665/341996/9789240029200-eng.pdf?sequence=1

[5] World Health Organization. Ethics and governance of artificial intelligence for health: WHO guidance executive summary [Online]. 2021 [cited 2025 Jan 22]. Available from: https://iris.who.int/bitstream/handle/10665/350567/9789240037403-eng.pdf?sequence=1

[6] Naik N, Hameed BMZ, Shetty DK, *et al.* Legal and ethical consideration in artificial intelligence in healthcare: Who takes responsibility? Front Surg 2022; 9: 862322.
[http://dx.doi.org/10.3389/fsurg.2022.862322] [PMID: 35360424]

[7] Sablone S, Bellino M, Cardinale AN, Esposito M, Sessa F, Salerno M. Artificial intelligence in healthcare: An Italian perspective on ethical and medico-legal implications. Front Med (Lausanne) 2024; 11: 1343456.
[http://dx.doi.org/10.3389/fmed.2024.1343456] [PMID: 38887675]

[8] Nasir S, Khan RA, Bai S. Ethical framework for harnessing the power of AI in healthcare and beyond. IEEE Access 2024; 12: 31014-35.
Available from: https://ieeexplore.ieee.org/document/10445375/citations#citations [Online].
[http://dx.doi.org/10.1109/ACCESS.2024.3369912]

[9] Oniani D, Hilsman J, Peng Y, *et al.* Adopting and expanding ethical principles for artificial intelligence from military to healthcare. Digit Med. 2023;225(6):1–10.
[http://dx.doi.org/10.1038/s41746-023-00965-x]

[10] Nuffield Council on Bioethics. Artificial Intelligence (AI) in healthcare and research [Online]. London: Nuffield Council on Bioethics; 2018 [cited 2025 Jan 22]. Available from: https://www.nuffieldbioethics.org/assets/pdfs/Artificial-Intelligence-AI-in-healthcare-and-research.pdf

[11] Raikes J. AI can be racist: Let's make sure it works for everyone [Online]. Forbes. 2023 Apr 21 [cited 2025 Jan 22]. Available from: https://www.forbes.com/sites/jeffraikes/2023/04/21/ai-can-be-rac-st-lets-make-sure-it-works-for-everyone/

[12] AI in the UK: Ready, willing and able? (Select committee on artificial intelligence - report of session 2017-19). London: UK Parliament 2018.

[13] Otto P, Graf E, editors. 3TH1CS: A reinvention of ethics in the digital age? iRights Media; 2017.

[14] Sharkey A, Sharkey N. Granny and the robots: ethical issues in robot care for the elderly. Ethics Inf Technol 2012; 14(1): 27-40.
[http://dx.doi.org/10.1007/s10676-010-9234-6]

[15] Gretton C. The dangers of AI in health care: Risk homeostasis and automatic bias [Online]. Medium. 2017 Jun 25 [cited 2025 Jan 22]. Available from: https://towardsdatascience.com/the-dangers-of-a--in-health-care-risk-homeostasis-and-automation-bias-148477a9080f

[16] Finlayson SG, Chung HW, Kohane IS, Beam AL. Adversarial attacks against medical deep learning systems [Online]. 2019 [cited 2025 Jan 22]. Available from: https://arxiv.org/pdf/1804.05296

[17] Milmo D, Farah H. Malicious use of AI could cause 'unimaginable' damage, says UN boss [Online]. The Guardian. 2023 Jul 18 [cited 2025 Jan 22]. Available from: https://www.theguardian.com/technology/2023/jul/18/malicious-use-of-ai-could-cause-huge-damage-says-un-boss

[18] U.S. Food & Drug Administration. Artificial Intelligence & Medical Products: How CBER, CDER, CDRH, and OCP are working together. 2024.

[19] Farhud DD, Zokaei S. Ethical issues of artificial intelligence in medicine and healthcare. Iran J Public Health. 2021;50(11):i-v.
[http://dx.doi.org/10.18502/ijph.v50i11.7600]

[20] Eslamitabar S, Lame E, Rouzbahani A, Roozbahani Z. Legal and ethical challenges of artificial intelligence applications in healthcare. Health Technology Assessment in Action 2024; 7(4): 1-5.
[http://dx.doi.org/10.18502/htaa.v7i4.14653]

[21] Gerke S, Minssen T, Cohen G. Ethical and legal challenges of artificial intelligence-driven healthcare. In: Artificial Intelligence in Healthcare. 2020. pp. 295–336.
[http://dx.doi.org/10.1016/B978-0-12-818438-7.00012-5]

[22] Sihlahla I, Donnelly DL, Townsend B, Thaldar D. Legal and ethical principles governing the use of artificial intelligence in radiology services in South Africa. Dev World Health 2023; pp. 1-11.
[http://dx.doi.org/10.1111/dewb.12436]

[23] Mohammad Amini M, Jesus M, Fanaei Sheikholeslami D, Alves P, Hassanzadeh Benam A, Hariri F. Artificial intelligence ethics and challenges in healthcare applications: A comprehensive review in the context of the European GDPR mandate. Machine Learning and Knowledge Extraction 2023; 5(3): 1023-35.
[http://dx.doi.org/10.3390/make5030053]

[24] Alberto IRI, Alberto NRI, Ghosh AK, *et al.* The impact of commercial health datasets on medical research and health-care algorithms. Lancet Digit Health 2023; 5(5): e288-94.
[http://dx.doi.org/10.1016/S2589-7500(23)00025-0] [PMID: 37100543]

[25] Liao SM. Ethics of AI and health care: Towards a substantive human rights framework. Topoi (Dordr) 2023; 42(3): 857-66.
[http://dx.doi.org/10.1007/s11245-023-09911-8]

[26] Belle V, Papantonis I. Principles and practice of explainable machine learning. Front Big Data 2021; 4: 688969.
[http://dx.doi.org/10.3389/fdata.2021.688969] [PMID: 34278297]

[27] Yang Z, Yu Y, You C, Steinhardt J, Ma Y. Rethinking bias-variance trade-off for generalization of neural networks. International Conference on Machine Learning 2020; 10767-77.
[http://dx.doi.org/10.48550/arXiv.2002.11328]

[28] Solanki P, Grundy J, Hussain W. Operationalising ethics in artificial intelligence for healthcare: A framework for AI developers. AI Ethics 2023; 3(1): 223-40.
[http://dx.doi.org/10.1007/s43681-022-00195-z]

CHAPTER 11

AI In Medicine and Healthcare Sector: An Analysis of Laws of Medical Negligence

Komal[1,*] and **Sagee Geetha Sethu**[2]

[1] *Department of Law, Gurugram University, Gurugram, India*

[2] *Amity University, Dubai*

Abstract: Artificial Intelligence (AI) is rapidly transforming the healthcare landscape, offering exciting possibilities from drug discovery to improved disease diagnosis and treatment planning. Real-world examples are woven throughout the paper to illustrate the significant impact AI already has on various aspects of patient care. However, implementing AI in healthcare is not without its challenges. Ethical considerations, data privacy concerns, and potential biases in algorithms are all critical issues that demand careful attention. The paper emphasizes the importance of transparency, fairness, and trust in developing and deploying AI-powered healthcare solutions. Obtaining informed consent from patients when AI is involved in their diagnosis or treatment is a complex issue that needs to be addressed. Ensuring the reliability and safety of AI algorithms, while maintaining transparency in the development process, presents another hurdle. Mitigating bias in AI algorithms is crucial to guarantee fair and equitable treatment for all patients. Finally, protecting patient privacy while enabling data sharing for AI development presents a significant challenge. Collaboration among healthcare professionals, AI developers, and policymakers is crucial to ensure that AI is used responsibly and effectively to improve healthcare outcomes for all. Beyond the potential of AI, the paper delves into the legal and ethical considerations that arise with its use in medicine.

The first aspect to consider is the copyright and patent rights associated with AI creations, as well as the question of liability. Can AI be held liable for medical negligence? If so, who is responsible – the AI itself, its creator, or some combination? These questions become even more relevant in the context of established medical negligence jurisprudence. This paper seeks to understand how different countries are approaching AI-based medical treatments and explores the prospects for future development. It also discusses the legal and ethical implications that may arise, analyzing the advantages and disadvantages of investing in AI for healthcare. By undertaking a doctrinal research approach, the paper critically evaluates the prospects of integrating AI into the healthcare sector and analyzes the policy and legal frameworks needed to ensure responsible use. This research is particularly relevant for policymakers and legal professionals responsible for shaping AI's future in healthcare.

* **Corresponding author Komal:** Department of Law, Gurugram University, Gurugram, India; E-mail: sandhukomal12@gmail.com

Neeraj Gupta, Abdelhameed Ibrahim, Bhavesh Vyas & Shobhna Jeet (Eds.)

Keywords: Advancements, Breakthroughs, Emerging challenges, Innovative technologies, Precision healthcare, Preventive care, Tailored medicine.

INTRODUCTION

Integrating Artificial Intelligence (AI) into healthcare has revolutionized medical diagnostics, treatment planning, and patient care. AI-powered tools, such as machine learning algorithms, robotic surgery systems, and predictive analytics, have enhanced precision, efficiency, and accessibility in medicine. However, the increasing reliance on AI in clinical decision-making raises critical legal and ethical concerns, particularly regarding accountability in medical negligence cases.

Traditional medical negligence laws are based on human error and professional liability, but AI introduces complexities where responsibility may be distributed among developers, healthcare providers, and even the AI systems themselves. As AI evolves, legal frameworks must adapt to address issues such as algorithmic bias, data privacy, and liability attribution in AI-related medical errors.

Individuals have rights and liabilities inherent to their liberty within society and under the law. These rights and freedoms are granted by the law and are supported by consequences for actions that infringe upon the freedom of others. The law aims to establish equilibrium in society by regulating the exercise of rights and imposing liabilities for any harm caused to others. The principles of liability arise from the interaction between the exercise of rights and liberties on one hand and the violation of the rights of others on the other hand. Intellectual property rights, too, are based on the concept of 'Balance of Rights' between the right holder and the interests of society. Both copyrights and patent law aim to incentivize the author/inventor of a new form of creation, which will, at the end of the term of protection, fall into the public domain, thereby serving to cater to the interests of the public. The IP laws are based on the premise of affording protection against any form of infringement, and hence, these are negative rights that grant a monopoly status to the right holder. The Utilitarian and the Labor theories are justifications behind the grant of IP rights, which seek to protect the rights and interests of the creator against any alleged infringer who tries to accrue unjust enrichment from the creations of the former.

The Law of Torts encompasses various civil wrongs, including negligence, which occurs when one person breaches their duty of care towards another person. This duty of care is imposed by law and requires individuals to take measures to protect, preserve, and respect the rights of others. Negligence can include reckless and careless behavior, regardless of whether there is an intention to cause harm. Recklessness occurs when someone is unaware of another person's rights and their duty of care. On the other hand, carelessness involves a lack of diligence and consideration for the potential consequences of breaching the duty of care. If a party is found negligent and their actions result in harm or damage to another person, they can be held liable for their actions and may be required to compensate the affected party. This ensures that individuals exercise their rights and freedoms without infringing upon the rights of others.

The concept of Artificial Intelligence (AI) and its applications in medicine and healthcare are explored in this article. It examines the potential implications of AI on copyrights and patents, questioning whether AI devices and their output should be eligible for intellectual property rights. Additionally, the article delves into the concept of professional and medical negligence, specifically focusing on cases of medical negligence involving AI. It discusses the legal framework surrounding the liability of doctors and medical practitioners and the importance of informed consent in determining their liability. The article aims to analyze the intersection of AI and tort law, highlighting the potential challenges and considerations that may arise in the future.

ARTIFICIAL INTELLIGENCE IN MEDICINE AND HEALTHCARE

R. Kurzweil has defined artificial intelligence as "the science of making computers do things that require intelligence when done by humans" [1]. AI can be defined as the capability of a computer program or a computer-controlled robot to perform tasks that would typically require human intelligence [2]. The Cambridge Dictionary has defined artificial intelligence as "the study of how to produce machines that have some of the qualities that the human mind has, such as the ability to understand language, recognize pictures, solve problems, and learn from experience". [3] Prolific developments made over a few decades in the recent past seem to have transformed the definition of artificial intelligence to 'an imitating intelligent human behavior'. [4] With the emergence of a new era, it is now possible for programs to generate original and novel creative works independently, without human intervention. Artificial Intelligence systems are designed to empower computers to perform tasks that typically require human-like intelligence [5]. AI systems are equipped with algorithms that learn from the data fed into them, enabling them to generate creative works with minimal human involvement. Artificial Intelligence is a field focused on developing computer programs capable of performing tasks that would typically require human intelligence, such as language translation and speech recognition. AI can be seen as the ability of a computer program or a robot to perform tasks that would usually require human intelligence [6].

The human mind has limitations, but Artificial Intelligence (AI) can perform countless calculations and make decisions indefinitely. AI consists of software and a learning aspect, where it develops through experience. It learns from various forms of input fed into the system. AI systems have certain inherent drives, such as self-improvement, self-protection, rational behavior, preserving utility functions, resource acquisition, and efficient utilization.

Creativity is no longer exclusive to humans. Self-driving cars, computer programs that generate artwork, creative machines, and learning algorithms have transformed the employment landscape in creative fields. As a creative machine, AI can imitate and replicate human neural networks using computer programming algorithms. It can operate with or without human intervention and even create new works of art, potentially replacing humans in the realm of creativity and innovation.

AI technology is advancing rapidly in the medical field. For example, GlaxoSmithKline has partnered with Exscientia, a British biotech company, to leverage its deep learning technology in the development of life-saving drugs. Exscientia's AI system analyzes molecular behavior to predict a drug's effectiveness, helping to reduce costs and discovery times by 75%.

Overall, AI presents opportunities and challenges across various sectors, including medicine and healthcare. Its potential to revolutionize industries raises questions about copyrights and patents for AI devices and their output. Additionally, the liability of medical professionals in cases involving AI and the importance of informed consent present legal considerations in the intersection of AI and tort law.

The medicine and healthcare industry has long relied on machine learning and decision-making processes. Many medical instruments, such as the pulse oximeter, ECG machine, pacemaker, blood sugar machine, and blood pressure measuring machine, can be considered forms of AI. These devices aim to simplify measurements and calculations that may be challenging for the human mind to complete accurately and within time constraints. The issue arises when people assign a more complex interpretation to AI. In practice, artificial intelligence results from computer programming and decision-making processes executed by industrial devices that operate independently, without external human assistance or intervention.

Healthcare industries worldwide are confronted with four key objectives: improving population health, enhancing patients' healthcare experience, improving caregiver satisfaction, and reducing the growing cost of care. These goals can be achieved by integrating AI-driven technology, which can assist healthcare systems in delivering better health and medical support to their populations. [7] Currently, there are two primary forms of AI-driven medical technology in the healthcare sector: one focuses on assisting with clinical decision-making, while the other is centered around imaging analysis [8]. Clinical decision support tools assist healthcare providers in making informed decisions regarding treatments, medications, mental health, and other patient needs by offering quick access to relevant information and research. In medical imaging, AI tools are used to analyze CT scans, X-rays, MRIs, and other images to identify lesions or findings that human radiologists might overlook. During the COVID-19 pandemic, several AI-driven diagnostic technologies were developed for testing and screening COVID-positive patients. In clinical trials, AI helps streamline the process of assigning medical codes to patient outcomes and updating relevant datasets, enabling faster and more efficient searches for medical codes. For instance, two IBM Watson Health clients found that AI enabled them to reduce their medical code search times by over 70% [9]. The University of Georgia is recognized for developing an artificial assistant that helps a wheelchair-bound, blind student navigate independently on campus. Additionally, a robotic nurse named Pearl supports elderly individuals in their homes and retirement facilities, walking at a pace that suits the patient's needs, maintaining patience, and providing 24-hour companionship without objection [10].

Robotic surgery is an advanced application of AI in medicine that reduces human involvement in surgical procedures. It utilizes automated robots to perform intricate surgeries with remarkable precision, flexibility, and control, surpassing traditional methods. A typical setup uses a camera and robotic arms equipped with surgical tools. The surgeon controls these robotic arms from a computer console, offering a magnified 3D view of the treated area. This technology transforms surgery by improving accuracy and enabling minimally invasive procedures.

ARTIFICIAL INTELLIGENCE IN HEALTHCARE: A BOON WITH ETHICAL CHALLENGES

The digital revolution has undeniably transformed the healthcare landscape. Artificial Intelligence (AI) is rapidly emerging as a powerful tool, promising significant advancements in disease diagnosis, drug discovery, and treatment planning. This paper explores AI's immense potential in healthcare while also acknowledging the ethical considerations that need to be addressed for its responsible and trustworthy implementation.

AI's Transformative Potential in Healthcare

AI's ability to process vast datasets, identify intricate patterns, and make faster, more accurate decisions has significant potential to enhance patient care. Here are some key examples:

[1]. Drug Discovery and Development: AI can speed up the drug discovery process by analyzing large molecular databases and predicting potential drug interactions, helping to reduce the time and cost traditionally involved in drug development.
[2]. Medical Diagnosis: AI algorithms can accurately analyze medical images, such as X-rays and MRIs, aiding in the early detection of diseases and improving diagnostic efficiency. AI systems, for example, have demonstrated promising results in detecting cancers and other abnormalities.
[3]. Treatment Planning and Personalized Medicine: By examining a patient's medical history, genetic profile, and lifestyle factors, AI can predict how they might respond to treatments, enabling more personalized and effective treatment plans with fewer side effects.
[4]. Robot-Assisted Surgery: AI-guided robotic surgery systems can enhance precision and reduce human error during complex procedures, leading to quicker recovery times and better patient outcomes.
[5]. Epidemic Prevention and Management: AI can analyze real-time data on disease outbreaks to predict and monitor the spread of infectious diseases, supporting public health interventions and improving outbreak containment.

AI is not just a futuristic concept; it is already making a tangible difference in healthcare settings. Here are a few recent examples:

- Atomwise and the fight against Ebola: In 2015, during the Ebola outbreak in West Africa, Atomwise, a company specializing in AI-powered drug discovery, collaborated with the University of Toronto and IBM to identify potential drug candidates for Ebola treatment. This rapid response through AI technology showcased the potential for faster treatment development during future outbreaks.
- AI-powered analysis of COVID-19 therapies: In 2020, AI was used to analyze the activity of dozens of medications and their ability to inhibit an enzyme crucial for SARS-CoV-2 replication. This research contributed to the development of potential COVID-19 therapies.
- IBM Watson for Oncology: This AI system, designed to assist in cancer treatment recommendations, received criticism for suggesting "unsafe and erroneous" treatment options. Concerns were raised about the limited and potentially biased training data used for the system.

- Royal Free NHS Trust and Google DeepMind: This case involved a data privacy breach. Patient data was shared with Google DeepMind without proper patient consent. This incident highlights the importance of transparency and patient autonomy in data sharing for AI development.

ETHICAL CONSIDERATIONS: NAVIGATING THE CHALLENGES

Although the potential benefits of AI in healthcare are clear, it is essential to address ethical considerations to ensure its responsible and trustworthy implementation. Here are some key challenges that require careful attention:

- Informed Consent: As AI plays an increasingly significant role in diagnosis and treatment, the traditional concept of informed consent becomes more complex. Patients need to understand how AI is being used in their care and how it may impact their decisions. For instance, how will patients be informed about the limitations of AI algorithms and potential biases?
- Safety and Transparency: The safety and reliability of AI algorithms are paramount. Training data needs to be robust and unbiased to ensure accurate and reliable outputs. Transparency in the development and use of AI is crucial for building trust with patients and healthcare professionals. Cases like IBM Watson for Oncology, which offered inaccurate cancer treatment recommendations due to flawed training data, highlight the importance of transparency and rigorous testing.
- Bias and Fairness: AI algorithms are susceptible to bias reflecting the data on which they are trained. If the data used to train AI systems is biased towards certain demographics, the algorithms may perpetuate those biases in healthcare delivery. For example, an AI system used for skin cancer detection might be less accurate for patients with darker skin tones if the training data primarily consisted of images from lighter-skinned patients. Mitigating bias involves carefully selecting training data and continuously monitoring AI systems to detect and correct emerging biases.
- Data Privacy: The large volume of personal health data needed to train and operate AI systems raises important data privacy concerns. Strong data security measures are crucial to safeguarding patient privacy and preventing unauthorized access to sensitive information. Striking the right balance between sharing data for AI development and maintaining patient privacy is a key challenge.

These ethical considerations are not merely theoretical concerns. Real-world examples illustrate the potential pitfalls of not adequately addressing them. The Royal Free NHS Foundation Trust case, where patient data was shared with Google DeepMind without proper informed consent, underscores the importance of patient privacy. Similarly, the controversy surrounding Project Nightingale, a collaboration between Google and Ascension to develop an AI healthcare tool, raises concerns about data ownership and potential conflicts of interest.

THE PATH FORWARD: RESPONSIBLE DEVELOPMENT AND DEPLOYMENT

The potential benefits of AI in healthcare are immense, but to fully realize these advantages, ethical considerations must be prioritized throughout the development and deployment process. Here are several key steps to ensure responsible AI in healthcare:

Collaborative Development: It is vital to encourage collaboration among healthcare professionals, AI developers, ethicists, and policymakers. This multidisciplinary approach ensures that AI is developed and utilized in ways that adhere to ethical principles and healthcare best practices.

Regulation and Oversight: Clear regulatory frameworks are essential for AI in healthcare. These should address data privacy, algorithmic transparency, and accountability concerns. Regulatory bodies must work closely with healthcare and AI industries to craft effective regulations that foster innovation while ensuring patient safety and privacy.

Human-in-the-Loop Approach: AI should complement, not replace, human judgment. A human-in-the-loop approach, where AI assists healthcare professionals without making final decisions independently, combines the strengths of both human expertise and machine capabilities. This ensures AI recommendations are thoughtfully considered within a patient's unique situation.

Education and Training: Healthcare professionals must be properly trained to use AI effectively and understand its limitations. Additionally, patients should be informed about how AI is being integrated into their care and what to expect. Building trust and ensuring transparency are essential for successful AI adoption in healthcare.

Continuous Monitoring and Improvement: AI algorithms must be continuously monitored and updated to maintain accuracy, reduce bias, and adapt to new information. Regular audits and evaluations are crucial for identifying and addressing any emerging issues.

By following these steps, we can ensure that AI is developed and deployed responsibly in healthcare. This approach will pave the way for a future where AI enhances patient care, leads to better health outcomes, and ultimately saves lives.

AI and Copyright Interface

Copyright Law is a branch of IP law that grants protection to the author or creator of a literary, dramatic, artistic, musical, and cinematographic work [11]. Literary works also include computer programs [12]. Copyright protects computer programs, which are defined as a set of instructions expressed in words, codes, schemes, or any other form, including machine-readable formats, that enable a computer to perform a specific task or achieve a particular result [13]. Protection is granted to the author of the computer program—the individual responsible for creating the work [14]. A computer program's source and object codes fall under the ambit of literary works under copyright law. However, the granting of copyrights for computer programs is governed by the AFC (Abstraction, Filtration, and Comparison) test in various jurisdictions [15]. Hence, several computer programs that have been developed to cater to finding solutions for a similar form of problem are excluded from the purview of being granted protection under copyright law [16]. AI is a software consisting of multiple computer programs that may form a protectable subject matter under copyright law. There are two aspects to granting copyrights to AI-driven technology or creations:

- One is where there is some human intervention involved in the creative or innovative process of AI. In this case, it is the author of the computer program who shall be accorded copyright protection.
- The other form of AI technology is autonomously generated creations or innovations.

In the second case, the question arises as to whether AI can be recognized as an author for copyright protection. The term author presupposes creations made by a 'person' using his effort, skill, and judgment. A person may be both legal and natural. However, in the case of an AI, attributing the status of a person to a computer program has not yet been dealt with under the jurisprudential definition of the term 'person'. Another limitation is that AI is driven by computer programming codes fed into its system by a computer programmer. Based on the coded algorithms, the computer program is configured to give certain specific output forms. For example, Alexa or Siri are designed and programmed in a way that they respond and give answers to questions for which the coding is already fed into their system. For example, questions like 'Alexa, will you marry me?' are never answered as the input of codes has not been configured to answer or respond to such questions. Another example is a 'weaving machine' that generates irregular shapes in fabric through a random process without identifiable patterns. Such creations are not eligible for copyright protection, as randomness is based on chance rather than creativity. Similarly, works produced by AI machines, where the human creator of the machine is not directly responsible for the outcome, would fall into the public domain. Hence, with the proliferation of AI-driven creations, technology will keep becoming more complex, requiring minimal or negligible human intervention. As a result, an increasingly autonomous creative process could leave many works without copyright protection. Therefore, copyright ownership and/or authorship in an AI-generated creation can only be attributed to a human being, in the legal sense of creativity and innovation.

AI and Patent Interface

Patents are granted to inventions that are proven as novel, non-obvious, and consisting of an advanced technological base, which may be used further for industrial application and usage. As per WIPO, "*a patent is an exclusive right granted for an invention, which is a product or process that provides a way of doing something, or offers a technical solution to a problem*" [17]. In terms of the form of protection, an AI-driven invention may be granted a software patent, depending on the utility and the functionality aspect involved in the said invention. In the case of Alice Corp. Pty. Ltd. v. CLS Bank International, the U.S. Supreme Court ruled that the patent in question, which related to a computer-implemented method for mitigating "settlement risk," was considered a mere abstract idea and therefore ineligible for patent protection under 35 U.S.C. § 101 [18].

However, under the Indian Patent Act and the TRIPS Agreement, the granting of a patent is prohibited for diagnostic and therapeutic equipment and instruments, which are crucial to providing diagnostic treatment, and is exempted. In fact, with the pandemic hitting the world, questions were being raised regarding the patenting of the vaccine for COVID-19. However, the widespread and immediate use of the vaccine for a massive population was considered more crucial, keeping in view the public health needs, than the prerogative of incentivizing pharmaceutical companies with patent rights, who had developed and invested huge amounts in inventing the vaccine. The question with respect to AI in the healthcare sector and patent law is whether or not patents should be granted to AI-operated or machine learning processes developed for therapeutic or diagnostic purposes. The simple answer to this question is that if the AI-operated device comes under suspicion of providing a therapeutic or diagnostic outcome, its eligibility for patent protection must be carefully examined. Another question, similar to the debate surrounding copyright and AI, is whether a new invention developed by an AI—if granted a patent—should be attributed to the original creator of the AI or to the AI itself.Further, in case the rights are vested, would it also have the right to sue and be sued? Most jurisdictions have opined negatively, as affording a legal personality to a machine may prove to be dangerous and against public policy and public interest in the long run.

MEDICAL NEGLIGENCE: JURISPRUDENTIAL ASPECTS

Negligence refers to a legally actionable failure to exercise the standard of care or skill expected in a particular situation, resulting in harm or damage to another person or their property. This breach of duty, whether through an act or an omission, occurs when someone does something a reasonable person would avoid, or fails to do something a reasonable person would undertake in similar circumstances. In negligence cases, the plaintiff must prove that the defendant owed them a duty of care, breached that duty, and caused injury or damage as a direct result.

Negligence per se is a specific legal doctrine in which certain actions are deemed negligent by default, eliminating the need to establish negligence based on the specific context. This typically applies when conduct violates a statute or a municipal ordinance or is so obviously reckless that no reasonable person would engage in it. A breach of a public duty established by law to safeguard individuals or property is generally classified as negligence *per se.*

Lord Macmillan observed, in Glasgow Corporation v. Muir [19, 20], that the actions of a reasonable person typically measure the standard of care in determining negligence. This standard considers both cautiousness and confidence, and it varies based on the circumstances of each case. Judges are tasked with deciding what a reasonable person could have foreseen in a specific situation and whether the defendant should have anticipated the potential for harm. If it is reasonable to foresee injury to the plaintiff, the defendant has a duty to prevent it, and failure to do so would make them liable. This duty to take care means avoiding actions or omissions that could likely result in harm to others. It is not enough to show that the injury was foreseeable; there must also be a reasonable likelihood of it occurring. Foreseeability does not imply likelihood; rather, the duty is to guard against probabilities rather than mere possibilities.

A professional is an individual with specialized knowledge or expertise in a particular field who offers services to the community. In their professional role, they are expected to adhere to a defined standard of care when dealing with others. Professional negligence arises when a professional either fails to take an action or takes an action that a competent professional in similar circumstances would not have undertaken. It reflects a lack of reasonable care, skill, or judgment and, in some cases, may involve intentional misconduct. In the medical field, such negligence can endanger the life or health of a patient.

In the case of Indian Medical Association vs. V.P. Shanta [21], the court established that professions possess four key characteristics, which are:

- Specialized Nature of Work: Professions involve tasks requiring specialized knowledge and skills, emphasizing intellectual abilities more than physical labor.
- Commitment to Ethical Principles: Professionals are expected to uphold ethical standards that go beyond basic honesty. Their responsibilities often extend to the broader community, sometimes outweighing their obligations to an individual client or patient.
- Professional Regulation: Professions are typically overseen by professional associations, which are responsible for regulating entry into the field and maintaining standards through codes of conduct and ethics.
- Medical Negligence: The courts recognize medicine as a profession, and any negligent act by a medical practitioner, hospital, or its staff is classified as medical negligence.

In summary, the court emphasized that professions are characterized by specialized skills, ethical commitments, and professional associations, and in the case of medicine, medical negligence may occur when a healthcare provider fails to meet the standard of care.

In the cases of Dr. Laxman Balkrishna Joshi v. Dr. Trimbark Babu Godbole and Anr [22], AIR, and A.S. Mittal v. State of U.P [23], the court established the specific duties doctors owe to their patients. These include:

- Duty of Care in Accepting a Case: Doctors must carefully evaluate whether they have the requisite expertise and resources to manage a patient’s case before agreeing to undertake it.
- Duty of Care in Determining Treatment: Doctors must make well-informed decisions about the treatment they provide, taking into account the patient's condition, medical history, and the available options.
- Duty of Care in Administering Treatment: Doctors must ensure the treatment is administered appropriately, precisely, and safely.

A breach of any of these duties may lead to a negligence claim. If a patient can demonstrate that the doctor failed to fulfill one of these duties and that this failure caused harm or damage, they may seek compensation.

The court also highlighted that negligence can take various forms, including active negligence, collateral negligence, comparative negligence, concurrent negligence, continued negligence, criminal negligence, gross negligence, hazardous negligence, active and passive negligence, willful or reckless negligence, and negligence *per se*.

Furthermore, in medical law and jurisprudence, a doctor's liability for negligence is not nullified merely by the patient's or their family's informed consent. While obtaining informed consent is a crucial aspect of medical practice, it does not absolve doctors from their overarching duty of care towards the patient [24].

Medical law evaluates the actions or omissions of medical practitioners using two primary ethical approaches:

- Consequentialism: This perspective assesses the ethical value of an action based on its outcomes. According to this approach, an action is deemed right if it results in positive consequences and wrong if it leads to negative outcomes. Often associated with utilitarianism, this view suggests that "the ends justify the means."
- Deontological Absolutism: This approach asserts that certain actions are inherently right or wrong, regardless of their consequences. It emphasizes duties and obligations, focusing on how best to fulfill them. From this perspective, the outcome does not always justify the means, and some actions may remain unethical despite potential positive results.

In determining a medical practitioner's liability for negligence, both approaches are considered. While the consequences of the practitioner's actions matter, their duty of care, adherence to medical standards, and protocols are equally crucial. Notably, obtaining informed consent does not absolve the practitioner of their responsibility to provide competent and reasonable care.

Liability and Informed Consent

Liability in medical law incorporates both the consequences of actions and the practitioner's duty of care. While informed consent is integral to medical practice, it cannot completely shield a practitioner from liability if there is a breach of their duty of care.

When it comes to the liability of a medical practitioner for negligence, both of these approaches are considered. While the consequences of an action are relevant, the duty of care towards the patient and adherence to medical standards and protocols play a crucial role in determining liability. Simply obtaining informed consent does not absolve a medical practitioner of their responsibility to provide competent and reasonable care.

In summary, in medical law and jurisprudence, the determination of liability for negligence of a medical practitioner involves considering the consequences of their actions; it also recognizes the importance of their duty of care and adherence to medical standards and protocols. Informed consent is an important aspect, but it cannot completely dilute the liability if there is a breach of the duty of care.

In the context of determining liability for the acts of a medical practitioner, the concept of informed consent is significant. Informed consent is a process that allows patients to make reasonable and informed decisions based on relevant information specific to their circumstances. It exists in two forms [25]:

- Express Informed Consent: Obtained through a signed consent form.
- Implied Informed Consent: Determined by evaluating the communication provided to the patient and whether they had a genuine opportunity to give valid consent.

There are also two perspectives on consent:

- Clinician-Centered View: This legalistic approach focuses on what the clinician must disclose to the patient about a procedure and its associated risks. It establishes a minimum standard to protect the clinician from liability.
- Patient-Centered View: This ethical approach prioritizes the patient's right to information, emphasizing what they need to make an informed decision. Commonly referred to as "informed consent," this view aligns with ethical principles.

Informed consent plays a crucial role in determining a medical practitioner's liability. It is a patient-centered process designed to provide the necessary information for patients to make informed decisions about their care. While both ethical and legal considerations are taken into account, the principle of informed consent is essential in safeguarding patient autonomy.

Medical consent is shaped by two contrasting approaches:

- Paternalism: This approach involves the doctor acting in what they believe to be the patient's best interests, even without the patient's explicit consent.
- Autonomy: This principle emphasizes the patient's right to make their own decisions, including the right to refuse treatment, based on the concept of bodily inviolability

In the legal case Sidaway v. Bethlem Royal Hospital [26], it was established that a physician meets their duty of care by providing sufficient information to enable the patient to make an informed decision. The extent of disclosure should align with accepted medical practices.

Informed consent requires ensuring that the patient comprehends the following:

- Nature of the Procedure: The physician should explain what the procedure entails and provide a straightforward description of how it will be performed.
- Risks Involved: Instead of listing every possible risk, the physician should focus on the most likely risks and those that the patient may find particularly concerning. If the patient inquires about a specific risk not initially mentioned, the physician must address it.
- Consequences: The physician should outline the probable outcomes of the procedure and discuss any potential alternatives.
- Alternatives: This includes explaining the likely consequences of not undergoing the procedure and providing information about other viable treatment options, especially if the patient expresses interest in them.

By ensuring patients clearly understand these aspects, healthcare providers can secure informed consent, uphold patient autonomy, and fulfill their duty of care.

For consent to be deemed valid [27], several key criteria must be met:

- Mental Capacity: The patient must have the mental competence to understand the information provided and make an informed decision.
- Voluntary Decision: Consent or refusal of treatment must be given freely, without coercion or undue influence.
- Adequate Information: The patient must receive sufficient details about the treatment, including its nature, risks, potential outcomes, and available alternatives.
- Voluntary Consent *vs.* Volenti Non Fit Injuria: It is important to differentiate between genuine voluntary consent and the legal defense of *volenti non fit injuria*, where a patient's acceptance of risks has specific implications.

The patient's willingness to accept risks plays a crucial role in validating their consent. The legal perspective on medical negligence differs between two main schools of thought:

- Tort of Battery: This view relates medical negligence to trespass against the person, focusing on cases where proper consent was not obtained. Here, the absence of informed consent invokes the concept of battery, highlighting the critical role of obtaining valid consent.
- Tort of Negligence: This approach treats medical negligence as a failure to exercise the expected standard of care. When disputes between doctors and

patients are addressed as consumer disputes, informed consent becomes a vital aspect of the duty of care.

In both perspectives, if a patient willingly accepts the risks associated with a medical procedure, negligence does not arise. However, if the patient is misled or inadequately informed about the risks, any resulting harm is attributed to medical negligence. This underscores the legal significance of providing patients with comprehensive information about potential risks.

Medical Negligence and Jurisprudence

In medical jurisprudence, practitioners can be held liable for negligence if their actions or omissions deviate from what a reasonable medical practitioner would do under similar circumstances. Courts assess liability by prioritizing the patient's life and health, weighing the risks and potential harm. If a practitioner's actions or omissions are found to be unreasonable and result in harm to the patient, they may be held accountable for medical negligence. In such cases, the court may award damages to compensate the patient for the harm caused.

In summary, valid consent requires the patient's understanding, voluntary decision-making, and sufficient information about the treatment. The legal obligation to provide adequate information about risks plays a critical role in determining liability for medical negligence.

The case of Bolam v. Friern Hospital [28] introduced the "prudent doctor test" to define the standard for determining a doctor's liability in cases of alleged breach of duty. Under this test, a doctor is not deemed negligent if their actions or omissions align with those of a reasonable doctor in similar circumstances. This approach was designed to shield doctors from undue liability.

In Canterbury v. Spence [29], the U.S. Court of Appeals introduced the "reasonable person standard," also known as the Canterbury principle. This principle requires doctors to disclose all "material risks" to patients to ensure that consent is truly informed. The court emphasized that genuine consent involves the patient's ability to assess the available options and their associated risks. Recognizing that the average patient may have limited medical knowledge, the court stated that it is the physician's responsibility to provide all necessary information to the patient to make an informed decision. The court also ruled that performing surgery without proper consent could be considered battery.

Maynard v. West Midlands [30] Regional Health Authority further emphasized the importance of doctors exercising ordinary skill in their appropriate specialty. It stated that a failure to do so by a specialist would be considered necessary for a finding of negligence. These cases highlight the importance of doctors providing reasonable care, obtaining informed consent, and exercising ordinary skill in their specialty. Failure to meet these standards can lead to liability for medical negligence.

Furthermore, in the case of Bolitho v. City Hospital & Hackney Health Authority [31], the courts ruled that if the professional opinion of a responsible body could not withstand logical scrutiny, the judge had the authority to deem it unreasonable or irresponsible and disregard it.

In the case of Chester v. Afshar [32], the principles of liability in medical negligence were redefined. It was established that when the duty to inform a patient is breached, the patient is entitled to a remedy. This led to the development of the principle of "implied causation" in medical negligence cases.

Montgomery v. Lanarkshire Health Board [33] further expanded the principles of liability in medical negligence. The ruling affirmed that patients have the right to consider their personal values and preferences when evaluating the risks and benefits of medical procedures, in addition to medical advice. The focus shifted from merely ensuring that sufficient information was provided for consent to whether the doctor acted negligently and upheld the patient's right to autonomy.

These cases demonstrate the evolution of the principles governing medical negligence liability, allowing for increased patient autonomy in decision-making and holding doctors accountable for breaching their duties.

In the case of Hii Chii Kok v. Ooi Peng Jin London Lucien and Anr [34], the court emphasized that the key issue was whether it was necessary for the doctor, according to the Bolam-Bolitho test, to obtain information from the patient through a proper examination. This focuses on the doctor's professional judgment, rather than the question of informed consent. As a result, the principles of liability continue to center on the actual actions taken by the doctor, which may be considered unreasonable by other professionals in similar medical emergencies.

Similarly, in an Indian case [35], the principles for determining the actions of a doctor are established through the development of tort law by the Supreme Court and High Courts. In the case of M/s Spring Meadows Hospital and another v. Harjol Ahluwalia [36], it was determined that in cases of medical negligence, Artificial Intelligence (AI) would be considered an agent of the hospital, and responsibility for any negligence would lie with the hospital or the doctor in charge, who would bear absolute liability.

Overall, these cases emphasize the continued application of liability principles in medical negligence, focusing on the actions of the doctor and the accountability of the hospital or medical institution involved.

The Answer to the Question of Liability

In the cases mentioned above involving AI and liability, the key issue is whether AI can be held responsible for its actions if granted certain rights. Liability is closely tied to rights, as every right carries a corresponding responsibility. However, liability can only be fulfilled by a person who can be held accountable. In the case of United States v. Athlone Indus Inc [37], it was determined that robots cannot be sued. Therefore, at present, AI machines cannot be held liable as they are considered either a product or a service.

The integration of Artificial Intelligence (AI) into the healthcare sector, particularly in diagnostics and therapeutics, raises profound questions about liability in case of medical negligence. This section explores potential scenarios to understand the complex interplay between human error, AI malfunction, and legal responsibility [38].

AI as an Innocent Agent

In scenarios where AI acts as a mere tool under human supervision, determining liability can be relatively straightforward. If the AI malfunctions due to errors in its programming or data input, the liability generally rests with the developer or the healthcare provider who failed to exercise due diligence in its implementation.

- Scenario 1: Malicious Programming: If the AI's actions are the result of intentional programming designed to cause harm, the developer would be primarily liable for criminal offenses. The healthcare provider who employs AI without due diligence may also face civil liability.
- Scenario 2: Human Error: If a healthcare provider inadvertently alters patient data, leading to incorrect AI output and subsequent harm, the primary liability rests with the healthcare provider.

AI as a Mistaken Agent

When AI makes errors due to unforeseen circumstances or limitations in its programming, determining liability becomes more complex.

- Scenario 1: Misdiagnosis Leading to Harm: If AI misdiagnoses a patient due to limitations in its training data or algorithmic flaws, the liability could potentially extend to both the AI developer and the healthcare provider. The developer might be liable for product liability if the AI's performance falls below reasonable standards. The healthcare provider's liability would depend on their reliance on the AI's output and the extent of their oversight.

- Scenario 2: Unintended Data Alteration: If an AI system inadvertently alters patient data, leading to harm, liability would likely rest with the healthcare provider or the AI's developer, depending on the circumstances under which the error occurred.

AI as an Autonomous Agent

The concept of a fully autonomous AI capable of making independent decisions raises even more complex liability questions.

- Scenario: Independent AI Malfunction: If an autonomous AI makes a decision that results in harm to a patient, determining liability becomes challenging. The AI itself cannot be held legally responsible. The developer might face liability if the AI's actions were foreseeable and preventable through better programming or testing. Alternatively, the healthcare facility that deployed the AI could be held vicariously liable under certain legal doctrines.

The allocation of liability in cases involving AI-assisted medical care presents a complex challenge with no straightforward solutions. As AI technology advances, the legal framework must adapt to address these emerging issues. Key factors such as the degree of autonomy granted to the AI, the transparency of its decision-making process, and the extent of human oversight will play a critical role in determining liability. A combination of strict product liability for AI developers, vicarious liability for healthcare providers, and potentially new legal structures for AI entities will likely be necessary to ensure patient safety and accountability in AI-driven healthcare.

The pressing need for a legal framework to govern AI liability is highlighted by the rapid development of AI technology, which currently operates in a regulatory vacuum. AI systems presently lack accountability for their actions. One potential solution is granting AI legal personhood or applying a common enterprise liability model to AI developers, users, and operators. However, it is also essential to establish robust safety standards, transparency protocols, and insurance mechanisms. A comprehensive approach encompassing these elements will be key to maximizing the benefits of AI while minimizing its potential risks.

CONCLUSION

India stands at a unique crossroads, poised to emerge as a global leader in AI for healthcare. Our nation's robust IT infrastructure, burgeoning startup ecosystem, and vast pool of skilled talent position us strategically. The government's emphasis on research and innovation, as evidenced by the National IPR Policy 2016, further strengthens this potential. However, realizing this vision necessitates a robust regulatory framework that balances innovation with accountability. Establishing clear guidelines for AI development, deployment, and liability is paramount. India has the potential to lead the way in developing ethical AI regulations, building trust and confidence among both patients and healthcare providers. By tackling the challenges of AI liability and ensuring transparency in AI algorithms, the country can cultivate a robust ecosystem for AI-driven healthcare solutions. This approach will not only enhance healthcare delivery but also establish India as a global leader in AI research and development.

REFERENCES

[1] TRIPS Agreement. Article 7, Objective Clause. 1994.

[2] Abbott, Ryan Benjamin, I Think, Therefore I Invent: Creative Computers and the Future of Patent Law. Boston College Law Review, Vol. 57, No. 4, 2016. [http://dx.doi.org/10.2139/ssrn.2727884]

[3] Artificial Intelligence Available from: https://www.britannica.com/technology/artificial-intelligence

[4] Cambridge Dictionary Available from: https://dictionary.cambridge.org/dictionary/english/artificial-intelligence

[5] Kok JN. Artificial Intelligence: Definition, Trends, Techniques and Cases. In: Encyclopedia of Life Support Systems (EOLSS). [Internet]. [cited 2025 Dec 4]. Available from: https://www.eolss.net/sample-chapters

[6] Gonzalez Otero B, Quintais JP. Before the singularity: Copyright and the challenges of artificial intelligence. Wolters Kluwer Available from: http://copyrightblog.kluweriplaw.com/2018/09/25/singularitycopyright-challenges-artificial-intelligence/

[7] Copeland BJ. Artificial Intelligence. Encyclopedia Britannica Available from: https://www.britannica.com/technology/artificial-intelligence

[8] Bajwa J, *et al.* Artificial intelligence in healthcare: Transforming the practice of medicine. FHJ 2021; 10: 1. [http://dx.doi.org/10.7861/fhj.2021-0095]

[9] IBM . Artificial Intelligence and Medicine. IBM Report 2020. Available from: https://www.ibm.com/topics/artificial-intelligencemedicine#:~:text=Artificial%20intelligence%20in%20medicine%20is%20the%20use%20of,quickly%20becoming%20an%20integral%20part%20of%20modern%20healthcare

[10] Hashiguchi M. The global artificial intelligence revolution challenges patent eligibility laws. J Bus Technol Law 2017; 13: 36.

[11] Stresing D. Artificial caregivers improve on the real thing. TechNewsWorld 2003.

[12] Indian Copyright Act, 1957. Section 13.

[13] Indian Copyright Act, 1957. Section 2(o).

[14] Indian Copyright Act, 1957. Section 2(ffc).

[15] Indian Copyright Act, 1957. Section 2(d)(vi).

[16] Whelan Assocs., Inc. v. Jaslow Dental Laboratory, Inc. (3rd Cir. 1986).

[17] Pai YA. Copyright protection for computer programs: Walking on one leg? J Indian Law Inst 2006; 48: 359-99. Available from: https://www.jstor.org/stable/i40163282

[18] World Intellectual Property Organization. Patents. Available from: https://www.wipo.int/patents/en/

[19] Rush S. The challenges of patenting artificial intelligence. Can Lawyer Available from: https://www.canadianlawyermag.com/news/opinion/the-challenges-of-patenting-artifi-ial-intelligence/274698

[20] Glasgow Corp v. Muir 1943] A.C. 448.

[21] Indian Medical Association v. V.P. Shanta. 1995 SCC (6) 651.

[22] Dr. Laxman Balkrishna Joshi v. Dr. Trimbark Babu Godbole and Anr. AIR 1969 SC 128.

[23] AIR 1989 SC 1570.

[24] Ivanović S, . Medical law and ethics. Acta Med Medianae 2013; 52: 67-72. [http://dx.doi.org/10.5633/amm.2013.0310]

[25] Bhakuni H. Informed consent to clinical research in India: A private law remedy. Med Law Int 2020; 20: 256-83. [http://dx.doi.org/10.1177/0968533220958185]

[26] Sidaway v. Board of Governors of the Bethlem Royal Hospital, 1985. AC 871.

[27] Carr C. Medical law and ethics. 2013. ISBN: 978-0-203-56824-8 (e-book)

[28] Bolam v. Friern Hospital Management Committee, 1957. 1 WLR 582.

[29] Canterbury v. Spence. 464 F.2d. 772, 782 D.C. Cir. 1972.

[30] Maynard v. West Midlands Regional Health Authority, 1985. 1 All ER 635.

[31] Bolitho v. City and Hackney Health Authority, 1996. 4 All ER 771.

[32] Chester v. Afshar, 2004. UKHL 41.

[33] Montgomery v. Lanarkshire Health Board, 2015. UKSC 11.

[34] Hii Chii Kok v. Ooi Peng Jin London Lucien and another, 2017. SGCA 38.

[35] Jacob Mathew v. State of Punjab. Appeal (crl.) 144-145 of 2004.

[36] M/s Spring Meadows Hospital and another v. Harjol Ahluwalia. Civil Appeal No. 7858 of 1997.

[37] United States v. Athlone Indus Inc. 746 F.2d 977.

[38] Wu W. Isaac Asimov's Robots in Time. In: Sullivan K Intellectual Property, Communication Etiquette and Artificial Intelligence 1993.

CHAPTER 12

Précision Healthcare: Advancing Patient Care Through Decision Tools, Wearables, and Ethical Considerations

S Adeeb Mujtaba Ali[1,*], **Safia Begum**[1], **Mohammed Aleemuddin Naveed**[2] and **Mohammed Naseeruddin Mujahid**[3]

[1] *Salar-E-Millat Sultan Salah Uddin Owaisi Central Research Laboratory for Cellular and Molecular Medicine, Princess Esra Hospital, Deccan College of Medical Sciences, Kanchanbagh, Hyderabad 500058, Telangana, India*

[2] *Department of Respiratory Medicine, Princess Esra Hospital, Deccan College of Medical Sciences, Kanchanbagh, Hyderabad 500058, Telangana, India*

[3] *Department of Otolaryngology Princess Esra Hospital, Deccan College of Medical Sciences, Kanchanbagh, Hyderabad 500058, Telangana, India*

Abstract: Précision healthcare is a revolutionary approach to medicine that emphasizes individualized treatment plans based on each patient's unique needs. This abstract delves into several aspects of précision healthcare, including wearable technology, sophisticated decision-making tools, patient care paradigms, and related ethical and legal issues. Précision healthcare transforms patient care through clinical, genetic, and lifestyle data by tailoring treatment plans to optimize benefits and reduce adverse effects. Modern systems must process complex decision-making information, like Artificial Intelligence (AI) and Machine Learning (ML) algorithms, to accurately and promptly inform healthcare decisions. With the ability to continuously monitor vital signs, exercise levels, and illness biomarkers, wearables have become essential components of précision healthcare. These gadgets make it possible to gather real-time data, improving early health anomaly detection and remote patient monitoring. Nonetheless, there are important moral and legal issues with applying précision medicine. Considering problems like patient consent for data use, privacy protection, and fair access to cutting-edge technologies is essential. Regulatory frameworks must change to promote innovation in healthcare delivery and guarantee adherence to ethical norms and data protection regulations. In navigating the complex legal and ethical considerations terrain, this chapter offers a thorough overview of the multifaceted landscape of précision healthcare, highlighting its potential to revolutionize patient outcomes through tailored treatments, cutting-edge decision tools, and wearable technologies.

[*] **Corresponding author S Adeeb Mujtaba Ali:** Salar-E-Millat Sultan Salah Uddin Owaisi Central Research Laboratory for Cellular and Molecular Medicine, Princess Esra Hospital, Deccan College of Medical Sciences, Kanchanbagh, Hyderabad 500058, Telangana, India; E-mail: adshireen@gmail.com

Neeraj Gupta, Abdelhameed Ibrahim, Bhavesh Vyas & Shobhna Jeet (Eds.)

Keywords: Decision-making tools, Ethical issues, Legal issues, Précision healthcare, Wearables.

INTRODUCTION

Précision healthcare, also called précision or personalized medicine, is a transformative approach to medical treatment and healthcare delivery [1]. It aims to customize healthcare decisions, practices, interventions, and products to individual subjects/patients or groups of subjects/patients, depending on their individual characteristics. These features/characteristics include genetic history/makeup, biomarkers, lifestyle, and physical environmental factors [2].

The core principle of précision healthcare is to move away from the traditional one-size-fits-all approach, which assumes that the same treatment or intervention will work similarly for everyone [3].

Instead, précision healthcare leverages advanced technologies such as genomics, big data analytics, and AI to tailor medical care according to each patient's needs [4]. This approach allows healthcare providers to predict more accurately which treatments and prevention strategies will be most effective and safe for each individual [5]. Key elements of précision healthcare include:

- Genomics and Molecular Profiling: Understanding the genetic and molecular basis of diseases to identify genetic makeup or genetic variations that can influence disease development, progression, and response toward treatment [6].
- Data Integration and Analysis: Utilizing large-scale data sets, including Electronic Health Records (EHRs), genetic data, imaging data, and patient-reported outcomes, to derive insights and make informed decisions [7].
- Targeted Therapies: Developing therapies that target specific genetic mutations or biomarkers associated with particular diseases, thereby improving treatment efficacy and minimizing side effects [8].
- Preventive and Predictive Medicine: Predicting disease risk based on genetic predispositions and other factors, enabling early intervention and personalized preventive strategies [9].
- Patient-Centered Care: This approach involves putting the patient at the center of decision-making and considering their preferences, values, and goals when developing treatment plans [10, 11].

Précision healthcare can revolutionize healthcare delivery through effective treatment, reduced adverse effects, and optimized resource allocation. However, challenges such as data privacy concerns, integration of complex data sets, and equitable access to these advanced technologies remain essential considerations in their widespread adoption. In summary, précision healthcare represents a shift in pattern toward more effective and patient-centric medical care, promising to improve outcomes and quality of life for patients across diverse populations.

PRÉCISION HEALTHCARE AND WEARABLE TECHNOLOGY

Précision healthcare leverages wearable technology to collect real-time, continuous data on an individual's health parameters. Wearable devices monitor various metrics like activity levels, heart rate, sleeping patterns, levels of oxygen, blood glucose, etc. Wearable devices include fitness trackers, smartwatches, and biosensors [12]. The integration of wearable technology into précision healthcare offers the following:

- Continuous Monitoring: Wearable devices offer healthcare professionals a real-time view and a comprehensive continuous stream of data, which is more precise than periodic check-ups [13].
- Personalized Insights: Data from wearables can be analyzed alongside other health information (like genetic data or medical history) to personalize treatment plans and interventions based on individual health patterns and needs [1].
- Early Detection and Prevention: Wearables can detect subtle changes in health metrics early, enabling early intervention and preventive measures tailored to individual risks and behaviors [14].
- Patient Empowerment: Wearable devices empower patients and give them access to self-health data, promoting self-awareness, adherence to treatment plans, and active participation in their healthcare decisions [14, 15].
- Research and Development: Aggregated data from wearables contribute to large-scale studies and research efforts, accelerating the development of new treatments, interventions, and healthcare innovations [16].

While wearable technology enhances the potential of précision healthcare, challenges such as data privacy, measurement accuracy, and integration into clinical workflows need to be addressed to fully realize its benefits in improving patient outcomes and healthcare delivery.

DECISION-MAKING TOOLS IN PRÉCISION HEALTHCARE

Decision-making in précision healthcare is supported by various tools and technologies that enhance the ability of healthcare providers to deliver personalized and effective treatments [17]. These tools leverage advanced analytics, genetic information, and patient-specific data to inform clinical decisions [18]. Here are some key decision-making tools in précision healthcare:

- Genomic Sequencing and Analysis: Genomic tools enable healthcare providers to analyze the genetics of the patient to recognize variations in genetic makeup that influence the progression of diseases, their susceptibility, and treatment response. This information helps in selecting targeted therapies and personalized treatment plans [19].
- Biomarker Testing: Biomarkers are indicators to measure biochemical mechanisms within the body. Biomarker testing tools allow for identifying and measuring specific biomarkers associated with diseases or treatment responses. This assists in predicting disease outcomes, selecting appropriate therapies, and monitoring treatment effectiveness [20].
- AI and ML: Algorithms of AI and ML analyze high-end data, including genomic data, Electronic Health Records (EHRs), imaging data, and patient-reported outcomes. These tools can recognize correlations and patterns that human analysis may overlook, providing insights into disease risk, prognosis, and personalized treatment options [21] .
- Clinical Decision Support Systems (CDSS): CDSS amalgamate medical data from the patient's medical knowledge and guidelines to assist healthcare professionals in making evidence-based decisions. These systems may suggest treatment options, alert providers to potential drug interactions or adverse events, and support personalized care plans based on patient-specific characteristics and clinical data [22].
- Predictive Analytics: Predictive analytics use statistics and AI to predict future implications and outcomes based on a patient's history. In précision healthcare, predictive models can anticipate disease progression, assess treatment response probabilities, and recommend personalized preventive measures or interventions [23].
- Remote Monitoring and Telemedicine: Remote monitoring tools and telemedicine platforms warrant continuous monitoring of the patient's health metrics and facilitate remote conferences with healthcare professionals. This technology enables proactively managed chronic conditions, detects health issues at an early stage, and adjusts the treatment cycle in a timely manner based on real-time data [24].
- Ethical and Regulatory Frameworks: Decision-making tools in précision healthcare operate within ethical guidelines and regulatory frameworks to ensure patient privacy, data security, and responsible use of genetic and personal health information. Bid ability with standards is crucial in maintaining patient trust and advancing the adoption of précision medicine technologies [25].

In conclusion, decision-making tools in précision healthcare empower healthcare providers to provide personalized, real-time data-based care that improves patient outcomes and treatment efficacy and optimizes healthcare resource allocation. Continuous technological advancement and integration of these tools into clinical practices are key parameters in realizing the maximum potential of précision medicine in transforming healthcare delivery.

PATIENT CARE PARADIGMS

Patient care paradigms encompass the evolving approaches and philosophies in healthcare that prioritize patient-centeredness, personalized treatment, and holistic well-being. These paradigms shape the delivery of healthcare, emphasizing empathy, communication, and collaboration among healthcare providers and patients [26]. Here are key aspects of patient care paradigms:

- Patient-Centered Care: This paradigm is patient-centric. When making healthcare decisions, it considers patients' values, preferences, and individual circumstances. It promotes shared decision-making between healthcare providers and patients to tailor treatment plans that are in line with the patients' needs and goals [27].
- Holistic Approach: Holistic patient care identifies that health is impacted by physical, emotional, social, and spiritual factors. It focuses on treating the whole person rather than just the disease, integrating mental health support, lifestyle modifications, and complementary therapies alongside medical interventions [26, 28].
- Personalized Medicine: It tailors healthcare to individual genetic profiles, biomarkers, and personal health data. It employs technologies such as genomics, biomarker testing, and predictive analytics to predict disease risk, select optimal treatments, and monitor responses to maximize treatment efficacy and minimize adverse effects [1, 9].
- Preventive Medicine: Preventive care paradigms focus on disease prevention and early intervention to maintain health and well-being. This includes promoting healthy lifestyles, routine screenings, vaccinations, and risk assessments to identify and mitigate health risks before they escalate into more serious conditions [29].
- Integrated Care: Integrated care paradigms emphasize collaboration among healthcare providers across disciplines and settings to coordinate seamless care transitions, enhance continuity of care, and improve patient outcomes. This approach is beneficial, particularly for patients with complex healthcare needs or chronic conditions requiring ongoing management [30].
- Empowerment and Education: Patient care paradigms promote patient empowerment through education, information sharing, and the development of

self-management skills. Empowered patients are actively involved in their healthcare decisions, better adhere to treatment plans, and achieve improved health outcomes [31, 32].

- Ethical and Cultural Sensitivity: Ethical patient care paradigms uphold principles of respect, confidentiality, and autonomy in healthcare decision-making. They also recognize and respect cultural diversity, ensuring that care is delivered culturally and sensitively, aligning with patients' beliefs and values [33].

Patient care paradigms evolve with advancements in medical science, technology, and healthcare delivery models. Embracing these paradigms fosters a patient-centric healthcare system that is responsive, compassionate, and effective in meeting the diverse needs of individuals and populations.

ETHICAL AND LEGAL ISSUES

Ethical and legal issues in healthcare are critical considerations that guide decision-making, policy development, and the delivery of patient care. These issues ensure that healthcare practices adhere to moral principles, protect patient rights, and uphold legal standards [34, 35]. Here are key ethical and legal issues in healthcare:

- Patient Privacy and Confidentiality: Healthcare providers are legally obligated to safeguard patient information and maintain confidentiality. Ethically, respecting patient privacy develops trust and initiates open communication between healthcare providers and patients [36, 37].
- Informed Consent: This is an ethical principle in which medical care providers undertake to inform patients about the related risks, alternatives, and benefits of the prescribed treatment or proposed procedures. Patients must voluntarily consent to medical interventions based on this information [38].
- End-of-Life Care and Euthanasia: Ethical dilemmas arise in decisions surrounding end-of-life care, including euthanasia and assisted suicide. Debates center on respecting patient autonomy, alleviating suffering, and balancing the principles of beneficence and non-maleficence [39].
- Resource Allocation: Ethical considerations arise in the fair distribution of healthcare resources, including organ transplants, vaccines, and access to expensive treatments. Legal frameworks often guide decisions to ensure equitable allocation while maximizing society's benefits [40].
- Genetic Testing and Privacy: Advances in genetics raise ethical questions about using genetic information to predict disease risk, select treatments, and conduct research. Legal protections safeguard genetic privacy and prevent discrimination based on genetic information [41].

- Healthcare Equity and Access: Ethical principles of justice underscore the need for an equitable approach to medical care services, irrespective of race, socioeconomic status, ethnicity, or geographical location. Legal frameworks aim to reduce disparities and promote healthcare equity [42].
- Professional Integrity and Conflict of Interest: Healthcare professionals must uphold ethical standards of integrity, honesty, and accountability. Conflicts of interest, such as financial incentives from pharmaceutical companies, can compromise patient care and require transparency and disclosure [43].

Navigating ethical and legal issues in healthcare requires collaboration among healthcare professionals, policymakers, ethicists, and legal experts. Balancing ethical principles with legal mandates ensures that healthcare practices uphold patient welfare, respect autonomy, and promote justice in care delivery.

CONCLUSION

Précision healthcare represents a transformative approach integrating cutting-edge technologies, personalized medicine, and ethical considerations to revolutionize patient care. By leveraging advanced decision-making tools, such as genomic sequencing, biomarker testing, and AI-driven analytics, medical caregivers can tailor a patient-centric treatment regimen based on their health/ medical data, genetic makeup, preferences, etc.

Wearable technology has a central role in enabling continuous monitoring and empowering patients to proactively take part in their healthcare management. These devices provide real-time data on health metrics, supporting the detection of health issues at an early stage and discrete interventions.

However, implementing précision healthcare is not without challenges. Ethical considerations like patient privacy, informed consent for genetic testing, and equitable access to advanced treatments require careful navigation. Legal frameworks must ensure that the use of patient data complies with regulations and protects individual rights.

In conclusion, précision healthcare holds vast promise in improving patient outcomes, enhancing quality of life, advancing medical research, and more. By embracing ethical principles, leveraging innovative technologies, and addressing legal complexities, healthcare systems can effectively harness the potential of précision medicine to deliver truly personalized and compassionate care to all patients.

ACKNOWLEDGEMENT

The authors would like to thank Princess Esra Hospital, Deccan College of Medical Sciences, and Owaisi Hospital and Research Centre.

REFERENCES

[1] Johnson KB, Wei WQ, Weeraratne D, *et al.* Precision Medicine, AI, and the Future of Personalized Health Care. Clin Transl Sci 2021; 14(1): 86-93. [http://dx.doi.org/10.1111/cts.12884] [PMID: 32961010]

[2] Stefanicka-Wojtas D, Kurpas D. Personalised Medicine—Implementation to the Healthcare System in Europe (Focus Group Discussions). J Pers Med 2023; 13(3): 380. [http://dx.doi.org/10.3390/jpm13030380] [PMID: 36983562]

[3] Strianese O, Rizzo F, Ciccarelli M, *et al.* Precision and Personalized Medicine: How Genomic Approach Improves the Management of Cardiovascular and Neurodegenerative Disease. Genes (Basel) 2020; 11(7): 747. [http://dx.doi.org/10.3390/genes11070747] [PMID: 32640513]

[4] Quazi S. RETRACTED ARTICLE: Artificial intelligence and machine learning in precision and genomic medicine. Med Oncol 2022; 39(8): 120. [http://dx.doi.org/10.1007/s12032-022-01711-1] [PMID: 35704152]

[5] Mathur S, Sutton J. Personalized medicine could transform healthcare. Biomed Rep 2017; 7(1): 3-5. [http://dx.doi.org/10.3892/br.2017.922] [PMID: 28685051]

[6] Institute of Medicine (US) Committee on Assessing Interactions Among Social, Behavioral, and Genetic Factors in Health; Hernandez LM, Blazer DG, editors. Genes, Behavior, and the Social Environment: Moving Beyond the Nature/Nurture Debate. Genetics and Health. Washington (DC): National Academies Press (US); 2006. 3, Available from: https://www.ncbi.nlm.nih.gov/books/NBK19932/

[7] Ehrenstein V, Kharrazi H, Lehmann H, et al. Obtaining Data From Electronic Health Records. In: Gliklich RE, Leavy MB, Dreyer NA, editors. Tools and Technologies for Registry Interoperability, Registries for Evaluating Patient Outcomes: A User's Guide, 3rd Edition, Addendum 2 [Internet]. Rockville (MD): Agency for Healthcare Research and Quality (US); 2019 Oct. Chapter 4. Available from: https://www.ncbi.nlm.nih.gov/books/NBK551878/

[8] Committee on Policy Issues in the Clinical Development and Use of Biomarkers for Molecularly Targeted Therapies; Board on Health Care Services; Institute of Medicine; National Academies of Sciences, Engineering, and Medicine; Graig LA, Phillips JK, Moses HL, editors. Biomarker Tests for Molecularly Targeted Therapies: Key to Unlocking Précision Medicine. Washington (DC): National Academies Press (US); 2016 Jun 30. 1. Available from: https://www.ncbi.nlm.nih.gov/books/NBK379335/

[9] Goetz LH, Schork NJ. Personalized medicine: motivation, challenges, and progress. Fertil Steril 2018; 109(6): 952-63. [http://dx.doi.org/10.1016/j.fertnstert.2018.05.006] [PMID: 29935653]

[10] Say RE, Thomson R. The importance of patient preferences in treatment decisions--challenges for doctors. BMJ 2003; 327(7414): 542-5. [http://dx.doi.org/10.1136/bmj.327.7414.542] [PMID: 12958116]

[11] Fisher KA, Tan ASL, Matlock DD, Saver B, Mazor KM, Pieterse AH. Keeping the patient in the center: Common challenges in the practice of shared decision making. Patient Educ Couns 2018; 101(12): 2195-201. [http://dx.doi.org/10.1016/j.pec.2018.08.007] [PMID: 30144968]

[12] Shajari S, Kuruvinashetti K, Komeili A, Sundararaj U. The emergence of AI-based wearable sensors

for digital health technology: a review. Sensors (Basel) 2023; 23(23): 9498.
[http://dx.doi.org/10.3390/s23239498]

[13] Vijayan V, Connolly JP, Condell J, McKelvey N, Gardiner P. Review of wearable devices and data collection considerations for connected health. Sensors (Basel) 2021; 21(16): 5589.
[http://dx.doi.org/10.3390/s21165589]

[14] Kang HS, Exworthy M. Wearing the future-wearables to empower users to take greater responsibility for their health and care: scoping review. JMIR Mhealth Uhealth 2022; 10(7): e35684.
[http://dx.doi.org/10.2196/35684]

[15] Mattison G, Canfell O, Forrester D. The influence of wearables on health care outcomes in chronic disease: systematic review. J Med Internet Res 2022; 24(7): e36690.
[http://dx.doi.org/10.2196/36690]

[16] Huhn S, Axt M, Gunga HC. The impact of wearable technologies in health research: scoping review. JMIR Mhealth Uhealth 2022; 10(1): e34384.
[http://dx.doi.org/10.2196/34384]

[17] Khosravi M, Zare Z, Mojtabaeian SM, Izadi R. Artificial Intelligence and Decision-Making in Healthcare: A Thematic Analysis of a Systematic Review of Reviews. Health Serv Res Manag Epidemiol 2024; 112333392824123486 3
[http://dx.doi.org/10.1177/23333928241234863] [PMID: 38449840]

[18] Alowais SA, Alghamdi SS, Alsuhebany N, *et al.* Revolutionizing healthcare: the role of artificial intelligence in clinical practice. BMC Med Educ 2023; 23(1): 689.
[http://dx.doi.org/10.1186/s12909-023-04698-z] [PMID: 37740191]

[19] Hassan M, Awan FM, Naz A, *et al.* Innovations in Genomics and Big Data Analytics for Personalized Medicine and Health Care: A Review. Int J Mol Sci 2022; 23(9): 4645.
[http://dx.doi.org/10.3390/ijms23094645] [PMID: 35563034]

[20] Bodaghi A, Fattahi N, Ramazani A. Biomarkers: Promising and valuable tools towards diagnosis, prognosis and treatment of Covid-19 and other diseases. Heliyon 2023; 9(2)e13323
[http://dx.doi.org/10.1016/j.heliyon.2023.e13323] [PMID: 36744065]

[21] Maleki Varnosfaderani S, Forouzanfar M. The role of AI in hospitals and clinics: Transforming healthcare in the 21st century. Bioengineering (Basel) 2024; 11(4): 337.
[http://dx.doi.org/10.3390/bioengineering11040337]

[22] Sutton RT, Pincock D, Baumgart DC. An overview of clinical decision support systems: Benefits, risks, and strategies for success. npj Digit Med 2020; 3: 17.
[http://dx.doi.org/10.1038/s41746-020-0221-y]

[23] Dixon D, Sattar H, Moros N. Unveiling the influence of AI predictive analytics on patient outcomes: A comprehensive narrative review. Cureus 2024; 16(5): e59954.
[http://dx.doi.org/10.7759/cureus.59954]

[24] Peyroteo M, Ferreira IA, Elvas LB, Ferreira JC, Lapão LV. Remote monitoring systems for patients with chronic diseases in primary health care: Systematic review. JMIR Mhealth Uhealth 2021; 9(12): e28285.
[http://dx.doi.org/10.2196/28285]

[25] Mennella C, Maniscalco U, De Pietro G, Esposito M. Ethical and regulatory challenges of AI technologies in healthcare: A narrative review. Heliyon 2024; 10(4): e26297.
[http://dx.doi.org/10.1016/j.heliyon.2024.e26297]

[26] Valizadeh L, Jasemi M, Zamanzadeh V, Keogh B. A concept analysis of holistic care by hybrid model. Indian J Palliat Care 2017; 23(1): 71-80.
[http://dx.doi.org/10.4103/0973-1075.197960] [PMID: 28216867]

[27] Edgman-Levitan S, Schoenbaum SC. Patient-centered care: achieving higher quality by designing care through the patient's eyes. Isr J Health Policy Res 2021; 10(1): 21.

[http://dx.doi.org/10.1186/s13584-021-00459-9]

[28] Tabish SA. Complementary and Alternative Healthcare: Is it Evidence-based? Int J Health Sci (Qassim) 2008; 2(1): V-IX.
[PMID: 21475465]

[29] AbdulRaheem Y. Unveiling the Significance and Challenges of Integrating Prevention Levels in Healthcare Practice. J Prim Care Community Health 2023; 1421501319231186500
[http://dx.doi.org/10.1177/21501319231186500] [PMID: 37449436]

[30] Geese F, Schmitt KU. Interprofessional collaboration in complex patient care transition: a qualitative multi-perspective analysis. Healthcare (Basel) 2023; 11(3): 359.
[http://dx.doi.org/10.3390/healthcare11030359]

[31] Vainauskienė V, Vaitkienė R. Enablers of patient knowledge empowerment for self-management of chronic disease: An integrative review. Int J Environ Res Public Health 2021; 18(5): 2247.
[http://dx.doi.org/10.3390/ijerph18052247]

[32] Bhattad PB, Pacifico L. Empowering patients: promoting patient education and health literacy. Cureus 2022; 14(7): e27336.
[http://dx.doi.org/10.7759/cureus.27336]

[33] Varkey B. Principles of Clinical Ethics and Their Application to Practice. Med Princ Pract 2021; 30(1): 17-28.
[http://dx.doi.org/10.1159/000509119] [PMID: 32498071]

[34] Haddad LM, Geiger RA. Nursing Ethical Considerations.StatPearls. Treasure Island, FL: StatPearls Publishing 2024. Updated 2023 Aug 14 Internet Available from: https://www.ncbi.nlm.nih.gov/books/NBK526054/

[35] Olejarczyk JP, Young M. Patient Rights and Ethics.StatPearls. Treasure Island, FL: StatPearls Publishing 2024. Updated 2024 May 6 Internet Available from: https://www.ncbi.nlm.nih.gov/books/NBK538279/

[36] Tegegne MD, Melaku MS, Shimie AW, et al. Health professionals' knowledge and attitude towards patient confidentiality and associated factors in a resource-limited setting: a cross-sectional study. BMC Med Ethics. 2022; 23 (1):26. Available from: https://www.ncbi.nlm.nih.gov/books/NBK9579/

[37] Tegegne MD, Melaku MS, Shimie AW. Health professionals' knowledge and attitude towards patient confidentiality and associated factors in a resource-limited setting: a cross-sectional study. BMC Med Ethics 2022; 23(1): 26.
[http://dx.doi.org/10.1186/s12910-022-00765-0]

[38] Shah P, Thornton I, Turrin D, *et al.* Informed Consent.StatPearls. Treasure Island, FL: StatPearls Publishing 2024. Available from: https://www.ncbi.nlm.nih.gov/books/NBK430827/

[39] Akdeniz M, Yardımcı B, Kavukcu E. Ethical considerations at the end-of-life care. SAGE Open Med 2021; 9
[http://dx.doi.org/10.1177/20503121211000918]

[40] Brock DW, Wikler D. Ethical Issues in Resource Allocation, Research, and New Product Development. In: Jamison DT, Breman JG, Measham AR, et al., editors. Disease Control Priorities in Developing Countries. 2nd edition. Washington (DC): The International Bank for Reconstruction and Development / The World Bank; 2006. Chapter 14. Available from: https://www.ncbi.nlm.nih.gov/books/NBK11739/

[41] Institute of Medicine (US) Committee on Assessing Genetic Risks; Andrews LB, Fullarton JE, Holtzman NA, et al., editors. Assessing Genetic Risks: Implications for Health and Social Policy. Washington (DC): National Academies Press (US); 1994. 8, Social, Legal, and Ethical Implications of Genetic Testing. Available from: https://www.ncbi.nlm.nih.gov/books/NBK236044/

[42] Williams JS, Walker RJ, Egede LE. Achieving Equity in an Evolving Healthcare System: Opportunities and Challenges. Am J Med Sci 2016; 351(1): 33-43.

[http://dx.doi.org/10.1016/j.amjms.2015.10.012] [PMID: 26802756]

[43] Institute of Medicine (US) Committee on Conflict of Interest in Medical Research, Education, and Practice; Lo B, Field MJ, editors. Conflict of Interest in Medical Research, Education, and Practice. Washington (DC): National Academies Press (US); 2009. Available from: https://www.ncbi.nlm.nih.gov/books/NBK22926/

SUBJECT INDEX

A

B

C

D

E

F

G

www.ingramcontent.com/pod-product-compliance
Lightning Source LLC
LaVergne TN
LVHW070951210926
848482LV00002B/173
* 9 7 9 8 8 9 8 8 1 3 5 3 6 *